CERTIFICATION EXAM REVIEW FOR DENTAL ASSISTING

PREPARE, PRACTICE AND PASS!

D0140532

MELISSA CAMPBELL
B.S., R.D.H., R.D.H.A.P.

CENGAGE
Learning·

Australia • Brazil • Canada • Mexico • Singapore • United Kingdom • United States

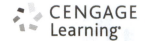
CENGAGE
Learning·

Certification Exam Review for Dental Assisting: Prepare, Practice and Pass!
Melissa Campbell

SVP, GM Skills & Global Product Management: Dawn Gerrain

Product Director: Matthew Seeley

Product Team Manager: Stephen Smith

Senior Director, Development: Marah Bellegarde

Senior Product Development Manager: Juliet Steiner

Senior Content Developer: Darcy M. Scelsi

Vice President, Marketing Services: Jennifer Ann Baker

Senior Marketing Manager: Erika Glisson

Senior Production Director: Wendy Troeger

Production Director: Andrew Crouth

Content Project Management and Art Direction: Lumina Datamatics, Inc.

Cover image(s): Photos from left to right: © Picsfive/Shutterstock; © Casarsa/istock-photo; © Tyler Olson/Shutterstock; Background: © rorem/Shutterstock

Unless otherwise noted, all items
© Cengage Learning

For product information and technology assistance, contact us at
Cengage Learning Customer & Sales Support, 1-800-354-9706
For permission to use material from this text or product, submit all requests online at **www.cengage.com/permissions**
Further permissions questions can be e-mailed to
permissionrequest@cengage.com

Library of Congress Control Number: 2015947175

ISBN: 978-1-133-28286-0

Cengage Learning
20 Channel Center Street
Boston, MA 02210
USA

Cengage Learning is a leading provider of customized learning solutions with employees residing in nearly 40 different countries and sales in more than 125 countries around the world. Find your local representative at **www.cengage.com**.

To learn more about Cengage Learning Solutions, visit **www.cengage.com**

Purchase any of our products at your local college store or at our preferred online store **www.cengagebrain.com**

Unless otherwise noted all items © Cengage Learning.

Notice to the Reader

Publisher does not warrant or guarantee any of the products described herein or perform any independent analysis in connection with any of the product information contained herein. Publisher does not assume, and expressly disclaims, any obligation to obtain and include information other than that provided to it by the manufacturer. The reader is expressly warned to consider and adopt all safety precautions that might be indicated by the activities described herein and to avoid all potential hazards. By following the instructions contained herein, the reader willingly assumes all risks in connection with such instructions. The publisher makes no representations or warranties of any kind, including but not limited to, the warranties of fitness for particular purpose or merchantability, nor are any such representations implied with respect to the material set forth herein, and the publisher takes no responsibility with respect to such material. The publisher shall not be liable for any special, consequential, or exemplary damages resulting, in whole or part, from the readers' use of, or reliance upon, this material.

Dedication
This text is dedicated to all of the dental assistants
who are committed to total patient care—and to Ron and Jordan,
without whose support this review would not have been possible.

Contents

Preface

The purpose of this manual is to assist you in preparing for the Dental Assisting National Board Examination or other dental assisting exam that you may encounter in your dental assisting career. Whether you are a dental assisting student preparing to take the Dental Assisting National Board Examination or a seasoned assistant interested in expanding your credentials, this manual will be an invaluable tool for studying and reviewing basic dental assisting information.

This review manual is arranged in an outline format to enable you to easily review dental assisting material that will be covered, and the end-of-the-chapter questions are available to assist you in further reviewing and testing the material. Whatever method you choose to study for any component of the Dental Assisting National Board Examination, the most important concept to keep in mind is that reviewing should be a way to refresh already-learned concepts. You should not rely on this review material alone to prepare you for the Exam. Instead, you should use several sources to study from. Be especially careful using the internet and make sure that you use trusted websites that will give you accurate information.

Study Techniques

When it comes to taking a test, we all get a little anxious. We wouldn't be human if we didn't. There is no substitute for knowledge. To pass a test successfully, you must simply know the material you are being tested on. However, there are some strategies that you can follow to help increase the probability of passing with a higher score.

1. Begin studying several months before the exam. Split the exam sections up in small parts and study them thoroughly one at a time. Don't wait until the night before to try and cram for the test but instead take that time to relax and get ready for the next day.
2. Use more than one source for studying. Research other review books, download the DANB blueprints for the exam from their website, dental assisting textbooks, reliable websites, flashcards, mock exams, and OSHA and CDC publications, are a few examples.
3. Wear comfortable clothes.
4. Eat something light before the exam, it is going to take you several hours to complete it.
5. Research your testing site and leave with plenty of time to get there, find a parking place, and find the testing location.
6. The exam will be presented with multiple choice questions. Exams are administered by computer. If you are uncertain how to use a computer go over the fundamentals with a friend or relative. Be sure to read the questions thoroughly before answering and try not to read into the questions. Attempt to answer the questions in your head before you look at the answers. If you cannot determine the answers with certainty eliminate the choices you know are incorrect.
7. RELAX. You know this information and you have prepared for the exam. Take your time and pick the best answer and unless you know with certainty that your answer is incorrect, try to refrain from changing any of your answers.
8. Bring a photo id and your test admission notice to the exam site. Do not bring children, friends, relatives, or spouses.
9. The DANB website provides a short video on what to expect the day of your exam. It is advisable to watch it so that you can anticipate what is going to take place the day of your exam.

Note:

DANB offers five national certifications: National Entry Level Dental Assistant (NELDA), Certified Dental Assistant (CDA), Certified Orthodontic Assistant (COA), Certified Preventive Functions Dental Assistant (CPFDA) and Certified Restorative Functions Dental Assistant (CRFDA). DANB offers these certification exams, as well as component exams. Each DANB certification is made up of component exams that can be taken separately or in various combinations. DANB also administers state-specific exams for certain states.

Acknowledgments

I would like to acknowledge and thank the following people for their valuable input.

Wanda C. Hayes, BSDH, RDH, CDA
Your Technical College
Rock Hill, South Carolina

Lea Anna Harding, BS, Ed.
Gwinnett Technical College
Lawrenceville, Georgia

Gabriele M. Hamm, RDA, CDA, CDPMA, AS
Husdon Valley Community College
Troy, New York

Deanna M. Stentiford, Ed.S
The College of Central Florida
Ocala, Florida

Also, I would like to give a special thanks to the team at Cengage:

Product Team Manager, Stephen Smith
Senior Content Project, Manager Jim Zayicek
Senior Art Director, Jack Pendleton
Senior Content Developer, Darcy Scelsi.

CHAPTER 1 – GENERAL CHAIRSIDE ASSISTING

The General Chairside component of the Certified Dental Assisting Examination consists of 120 multiple-choice items. There are seven content areas of focus in this component of the DANB examination. These content areas are:

- Collection and Recording of Clinical Data (10% or 12 questions)
- Chairside Dental Procedures (45% or 54 questions)
- Chairside Dental Materials (Preparation, Manipulation, and Application) (9% or 11 questions)
- Lab Materials and Procedures (4% or 5 questions)
- Patient Education and Oral Health Management (10% or 12 questions)
- Prevention and Management of Emergencies (12% or 15 questions)
- Office Operations (10% or 12 questions)

It is anticipated that this component of the examination will take 1½ hours to complete. This chapter provides an outline and review of the testing topics and objectives on the General Chairside component of the DANB examination.

Section I:
Collection and Recording
of Clinical Data

This section of the General Chairside portion of the Certified Dental Assisting Examination consists of 10% or 12 questions of the 120 multiple-choice items. The questions related to this section of the General Chairside Dental Assisting Examination are based upon your knowledge of the following:

- Basic oral anatomy, physiology, and structures of the oral cavity
- The preliminary patient examination
- Dental charting
- Diagnostic aids
- Treatment documentation

Key Terms

cranial bones – bones that make up the skull

cranial nerves – innervation of the structures in the head

deciduous dentition – first set of teeth; not permanent

dental history – recording of the treatments and procedures related to a patient

frenum – raised lines of mucosal tissue found in the vestibule areas of the oral cavity

hard palate – anterior portion of the roof of the mouth

masticatory mucosa – tissue that covers areas of stress in the oral cavity

medical history – history of medical conditions and treatments of a particular patient

lining mucosa – tissue that covers all areas of the oral cavity

lymph nodes – structures found along lymph vessels; filter lymph as it moves back into the blood and manufactures antibodies for immune processed

soft palate – posterior portion of the roof of the mouth

Quick Review Outline

I. Collection and Recording of Clinical Data

  A. The dental assistant should demonstrate an understanding of the anatomy, physiology, and development of the head and oral cavity.

    1. Bones

      a. **Cranial bones**. There are eight bones of the cranium (Figure 1-1).

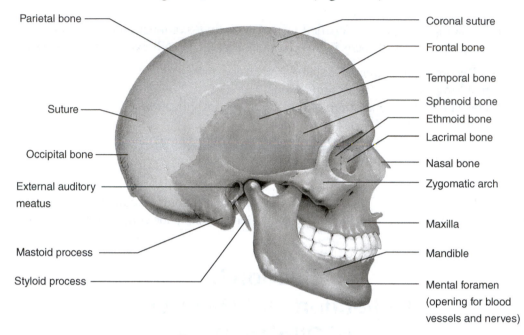

Figure 1-1 Bones of the cranium

        i. occipital (1)   iii. frontal (1)   v. ethmoid (1)

        ii. parietal (2)   iv. temporal (2)   vi. sphenoid (1)

      b. Facial bones. There are 14 bones of the face (Figure 1-2).

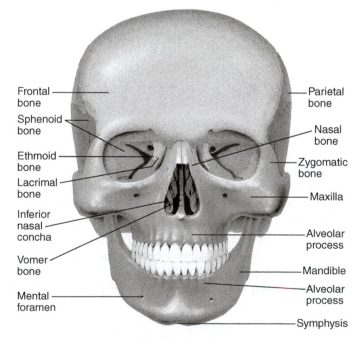

Figure 1-2 Bones of the face

    i. inferior nasal conchae (2)
   ii. vomer (1)
  iii. lacrimal (2)
   iv. zygomatic (2)

   v. palatine (2)
  vi. mandible (1)
 vii. maxilla (2)
viii. nasal (2)

  c. Types of bone (osseous) tissue. There are two types.

      i. Cancellous bone, synonymous with trabecular bone or spongy bone. It has a higher surface area and is less dense, softer, weaker, and less stiff but highly vascular.

     ii. Compact bone, synonymous with cortical bone. As its name implies, cortical bone forms the cortex, or outer shell, of most bones. Compact bone is much denser than cancellous bone.

2. Muscles

  a. Muscles of mastication (origin, insertion, and innervation) (Figure 1-3)

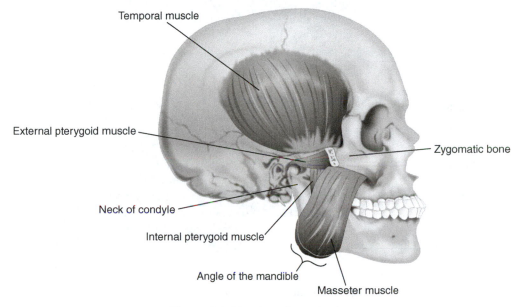

Figure 1-3 Muscles of mastication

      i. temporalis muscle

        origin: temporal fossa of the temporal bone

        insertion: coronoid process and the anterior border of the ramus of the mandible

        innervation: mandibular division of trigeminal nerve

     ii. masseter muscle

        origin: The superficial part originates from the lower border of the zygomatic arch. The deep part originates from the posterior and medial side of the zygomatic arch.

        insertion: The superficial part inserts on the angle and lower lateral side of the ramus of the mandible. The deep part inserts into the upper lateral ramus and coronoid process of the mandible.

        innervation: mandibular division of trigeminal nerve

    iii. internal pterygoid (medial)

        origin: the medial surface of the lateral pterygoid plate of the sphenoid bone, the palatine bone, and the tuberosity of the maxillary bone

        insertion: the inner surface of the ramus and angle of the mandible

        innervation: mandibular division of trigeminal nerve

     iv. external pterygoid (lateral)

        origin: the medial surface of the lateral pterygoid plate of the sphenoid bone, the palatine bone, and the tuberosity of the maxillary bone *insertion:* into the inner surface of the ramus and angle of the mandible

innervation: mandibular division of trigeminal nerve

b. Muscles of facial expression (origin, insertion, and innervation) (Figure 1-4)

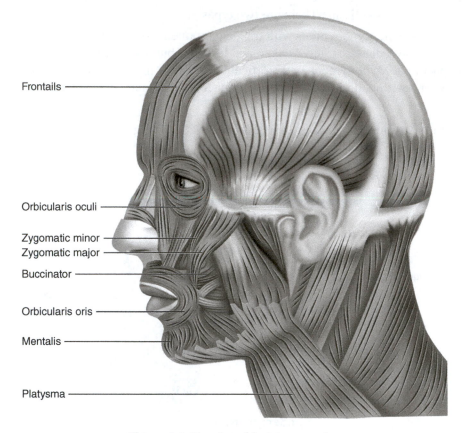

Frontails

Orbicularis oculi

Zygomatic minor
Zygomatic major

Buccinator

Orbicularis oris

Mentalis

Platysma

Figure 1-4 Muscles of facial expression

   i. Frontalis muscle: raises eyebrows and wrinkles forehead.

   origin: tissues of the scalp

   insertion: skin around eyes and eyebrows

   innervation: temporal branch of the facial nerve

  ii. Orbicularis oculi: the muscle that encircles the eye and is responsible for blinking, squinting, and forceful closing of the eyelids

   origin: around the eye

   insertion: around the eye

   innervation: zygomatic and frontal branches of the facial nerve

 iii. orbicularis oris: the muscle which circles the mouth and closes and protrudes the lips. The "kissing" muscle.

   origin: muscle fibers around the mouth

   insertion: skin surrounding the mouth

   innervation: facial nerve

 iv. platysma: depresses the mandible, draws angle of mouth downward, and tightens skin of the neck.

   origin: skin over lower neck and upper chest

   insertion: lower border of the mandible, mouth skin, and muscle

   innervation: cranial branch of the facial nerve

     v. buccinator: flattens the cheek and retracts the angle of the mouth.

       origin: alveolar process of the maxilla and mandible and the pterygomandibular raphe

       insertion: corners of the mouth

       innervation: buccal branch of facial nerve

    vi. mentalis: wrinkles the end of the chin

       origin: incisive fossa of the mandible

       insertion: corners of the mouth

       innervation: mandibular branch of facial nerve

   vii. zygomatic major: draws the upper lip backward, upward, and outward.

       origin: zygomatic bone

       insertion: angle of the mouth

       innervation: buccal branch of facial nerve

3. Glands and Lymphatics

  a. Salivary glands and ducts (Figure 1-5)

    i. Parotid: Located near the ear, this gland is the largest of the salivary glands. It secretes serous (clear liquid) substance.

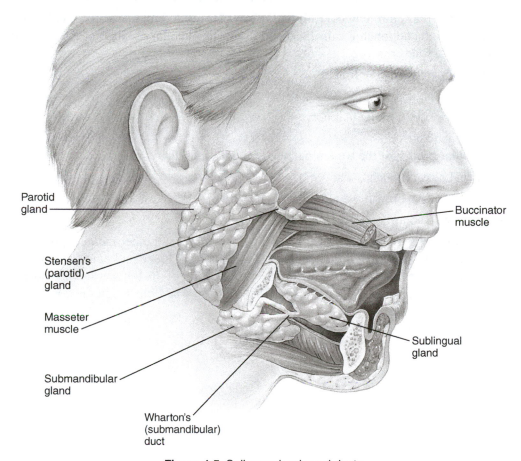

Figure 1-5 Salivary glands and ducts

Duct: Stensen's
    ii. Sublingual: Located under the tongue. This gland secretes primarily mucus (slimy glue-like substance). It is almond shaped and sits on either side of the base of the tongue.

Ducts: Rivinus and Bartholin's ducts attach to the sublingual glands.
    iii. Submandibular: Located on each side of the face. These are irregular in shape and secrete both serous as well as mucus secretions.

Duct: Wharton's duct is the duct that attaches to the submandibular gland.

  b. Lymphatics – system that drains and filters tissue fluid surrounding cells
    i. lymph – clear liquid found in tissue spaces
    ii lymph vessels – thin-walled capillaries that allow lymph to flow through body
    iii. **lymph nodes** – structures found along lymph vessels; filter lymph as it moves back into the blood and manufactures antibodies for immune processes
    iv. spleen – organ that removes bacteria and foreign matter from blood, produces and filters red blood cells and stores blood
    v. thymus gland – gland that develops lymphocytes and protects body from disease
    vi. tonsils – lymph tissues that guard against bacteria that may enter the body through the digestive or respiratory tracts

  4. Nerves
    a. **Cranial nerves**. Four cranial nerves innervate the face and oral cavity (Figure 1-6A and C).
      i. Trigeminal: plays a role in controlling the muscles needed for chewing and also provides the senses of pain and touch for the head and face. The maxillary branch of the trigeminal nerve divides into four branches:

- Pterygopalatine nerve branch
- Infraorbital nerve
- Posterior superior alveolar nerve
- Zygomatic nerve

The mandibular branch of the trigeminal nerve divides into three branches:

- Buccal nerve branch
- Lingual nerve branch
- Inferior alveolar nerve branch

      ii. Facial: Controls the muscles used in smiling, frowning, and other facial expressions. It also produces taste in two thirds of the tongue and sensations of touch and pain from the ear.
      iii. Glossopharyngeal: allows for taste on the back portion of the tongue and provides the sensations of pain and touch from the tongue and tonsils and also participates in the control of muscles used during swallowing.
      iv. Hypoglossal: allows the tongue to move properly.

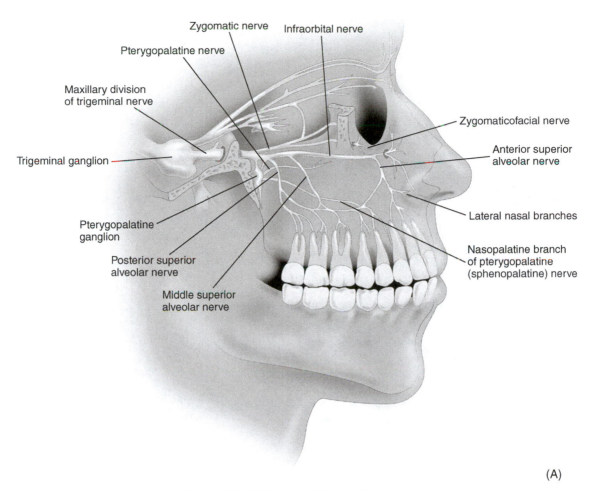

Figure 1-6 (A) Nerves of the maxillary arch

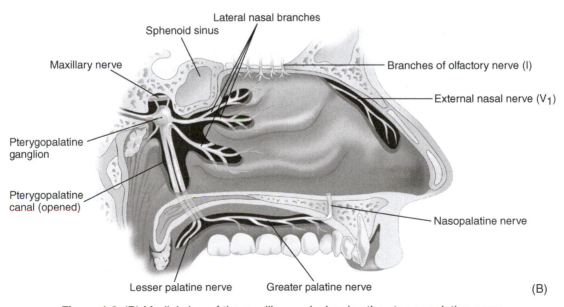

Figure 1-6 (B) Medial view of the maxillary arch showing the pterygopalatine nerve

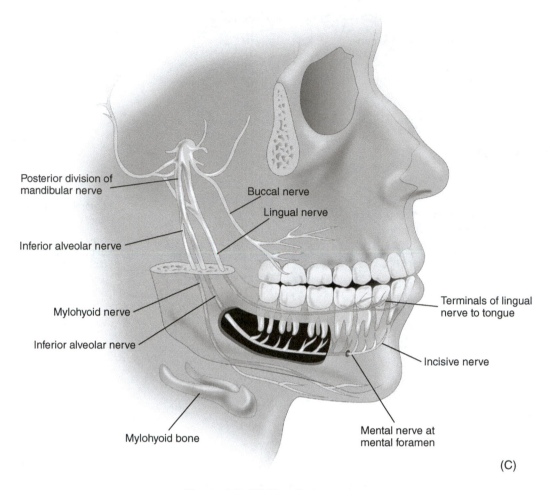

Posterior division of
mandibular nerve

Buccal nerve

Lingual nerve

Inferior alveolar nerve

Mylohyoid nerve

Inferior alveolar nerve

Terminals of lingual
nerve to tongue

Incisive nerve

Mylohyoid bone

Mental nerve at
mental foramen

(C)

Figure 1-6 (C) Mandibular nerves

5. Blood vessels
   a. Arteries (main branches) (Figure 1-7)
      i. The brachiocephalic artery is the largest artery that branches to form the right common carotid artery and the right subclavian artery. This artery provides blood to the right portion of the chest, arm, neck, and head.
      ii. Left common carotid artery divides to form the internal carotid artery and an external carotid artery. These arteries supply the brain, neck, and face.

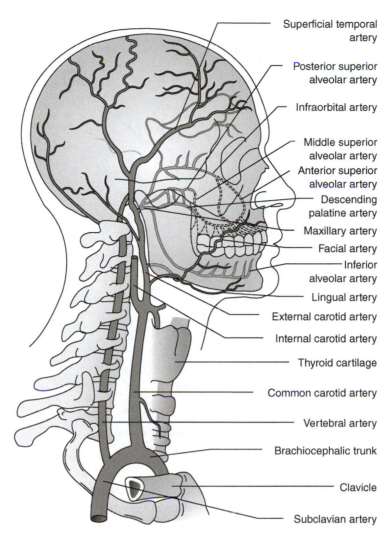

Superficial temporal
artery

Posterior superior
alveolar artery

Infraorbital artery

Middle superior
alveolar artery

Anterior superior
alveolar artery

Descending
palatine artery

Maxillary artery

Facial artery

Inferior
alveolar artery

Lingual artery

External carotid artery

Internal carotid artery

Thyroid cartilage

Common carotid artery

Vertebral artery

Brachiocephalic trunk

Clavicle

Subclavian artery

Figure 1-7 Arteries of the face and oral cavity

b. Veins (main branches) (Figure 1-8)

   i. Right and left internal jugular veins drain deoxygenated blood from the brain and neck.

  ii. Right and left external jugular veins drain deoxygenated blood from the parotid glands, facial muscles, and scalp into the subclavian veins, which flow to the superior vena cava and back to the heart.

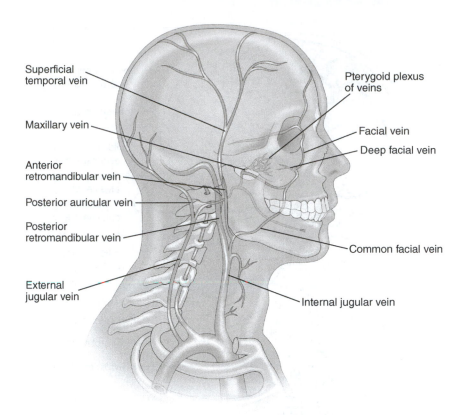

Superficial
temporal vein

Pterygoid plexus
of veins

Maxillary vein

Facial vein

Deep facial vein

Anterior
retromandibular vein

Posterior auricular vein

Posterior
retromandibular vein

Common facial vein

External
jugular vein

Internal jugular vein

Figure 1-8 Veins of the face and oral cavity

6. Teeth (Figure 1-9)

a. primary or **deciduous dentition**: The teeth lettered A–T, starting on the upper right. All are usually present by the age of 2. The primary dentition does not contain third molars or bicuspids.

b. permanent dentition: The teeth numbered 1–32, beginning with the upper right third molar and extending to the third molar on the left then dropping down to the third molar on the lower left and ending with the third molar on the lower right.

c. Divisions of the tooth

    i. anatomical crown – portion of tooth covered with enamel
    ii. anatomical root – portion of tooth covered with cementum
    iii. clinical crown – portion of crown that is visible in the mouth
    iv. clinical root – portion of the root seen in the oral cavity

d. Tooth Structure

    i. dentin – makes up the bulk of the tooth structures located around the pulp cavity and under the enamel within the anatomical crown and under the cementum within the root
    ii. enamel – tooth structure that covers the outside of the crown of the tooth
    iii. cementum – the tooth structure that is located around the root, covering the dentin on the root portion of the tooth
    iv. pulp – vascular and nerve network of fleshy connective tissue that fills the center of the tooth in the cavity formed by the dentin

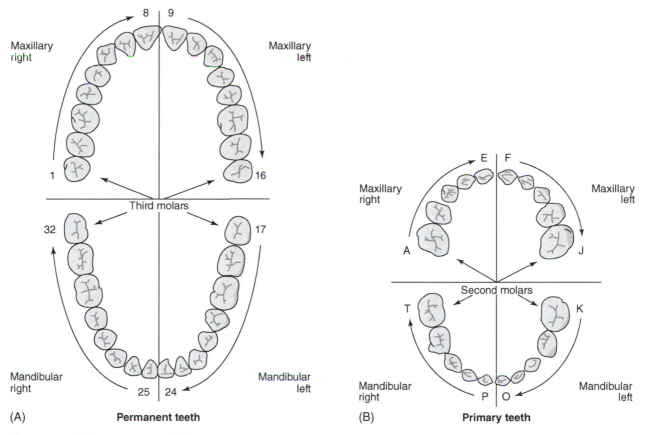

Figure 1-9 (A) Permanent and (B) primary dentition showing the Universal/National numbering and lettering system

7. Structures of the oral cavity
   a. Oral mucosa and gingival tissue
      i. **Masticatory mucosa**, which covers the areas subject to stress.
      ii. Specialized mucosa, which covers the area that covers the dorsum of the tongue.
      iii. **Lining mucosa**, which covers all other areas of the oral cavity.
   b. Attached gingiva, which is firm and dense and is bound down to the underlining periosteum, tooth, and bone.
   c. Free gingiva is the unattached portion that encircles the tooth and forms the sulcus, which surrounds the neck of the tooth.
   d. **Hard palate** is the bony anterior two thirds of the palate that is covered with keratinized tissue.
   e. **Soft palate** is the posterior third of the palate covered with mucosal tissue.
   f. Uvula is the pendent fleshy mass that is suspended in the back of the throat. Its function is not clearly known.
   g. **Frenum** (there are three types)
      i. Buccal frenum: the fold of tissue attaching the cheek to the alveolar ridge near the second premolar.
      ii. Labial frenum: the fold of tissue attaching the lip to the alveolar ridge near the midline.
      iii. Lingual frenum: the fold of tissue attaching the tongue to the floor of the mouth.
   h. Tongue is the muscular organ that aids in speech and prepares food for digestion.
      i. Circumvallate papillae: Formed into a V-shaped arrangement on the back of the tongue; appear relatively large and are where the "taste buds" are located. They contain taste pores with sensitive hair-like structures called microvilli. This is where the taste receptor cells are located.

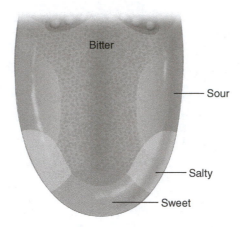

Bitter

Sour

Salty

Sweet

Figure 1-10 The location of the basic taste buds of the tongue

    ii. Fungiform papillae: mushroom-shaped papillae on the tongue. Aid in distinguishing the four tastes: sweet, sour, bitter, and salty (Figure 1-10).

    iii. Foliate papillae: Clustered into two groups on each side of the tongue, these papillae are involved in the sensation of taste and have taste buds embedded into their surfaces.

    iv. Filiform papillae: These small prominences on the surface of the tongue are thin and do not contain taste buds but instead are involved in a protective mechanism and is not part of gustation (the act of eating).

  i. Rugae are the ridges located on the anterior portion of the palate. The irregular surface is thought to aid in speech and swallowing.

  j. Palatine raphe is the visible "seam" in the middle of the hard palate.

  k. Tonsils (Figure 1-11)

    i. nasopharyngeal: also called adenoids, lymphoepithelial tissue which can be seen in the back of the throat on the roof of the pharynx

    ii. lingual: nonkeratinized tissue located at the sides of the oropharynx between palatoglossal and palatopharyngeal arches

    iii. palatine: nonkeratinized tissue located behind the tongue

B. Preliminary Examination: Understanding the preliminary examination means being able to review and interpret the patient's **medical history** and **dental history**. The assistant must listen to the patient and record his or her concerns with a high degree of accuracy.

  1. Recording patient chief complaints and relaying your findings to the dentist is part of understanding the preliminary examination.

    a. Being able to take an accurate medical/dental history is key because it enables the dentist to correctly diagnose and treat the patient to the best of his/her abilities.

    b. The dental assistant should be able to identify the key items to look for on the medical/dental history:

      i. any drug allergies or history of drug abuse

      ii. any antibiotic coverage for past surgeries or medical conditions

      iii. does the patient have a history of any communicable diseases?

      iv. are there any diseases with related oral manifestations listed?

      v. whether the patient is pregnant

      vi. any history of psychological disorders

      vii. any history of recent surgeries and medications being taken

      viii. any current illnesses and how the patient is being treated

      ix. primary physician contact information

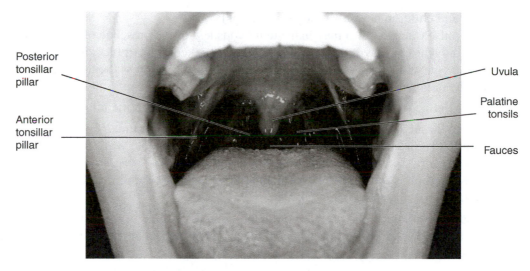

Posterior tonsillar pillar

Anterior tonsillar pillar

Uvula

Palatine tonsils

Fauces

Figure 1-11 Location of the tonsils

2. The dental assistant should be able to assess the patient's general physical condition and note any abnormalities.

   a. skin: note condition, variations in color and tone, damage, etc.

   b. gait: note any imbalance or incoordination

   c. abnormal characteristics: symmetry, speech impairment, hearing impairment, mannerisms

   d. evidence of eating disorders: below- or above-average body weight, skin condition, erosion of tooth enamel, brittle nails, thinning hair, impaired organ function

   e. evidence of substance abuse or physical abuse: bruising in different stages of healing, signs of trauma, patterns of bruising, tolerance or dependence on a drug

   f. age-related changes: changes in skin integrity, loss of sensation, loss of taste, loss of dexterity, hearing or vision changes

3. Demonstrate an understanding of how to take, record, and measure vital signs.

   a. Pulse is defined as a rhythmical beating of the arteries as blood is propelled through the blood vessels.

      i. A normal pulse is between 60 and 100 beats per minute (bpm).

      ii. The pulse is most frequently felt at the radial artery on the wrist (Figure 1-12).

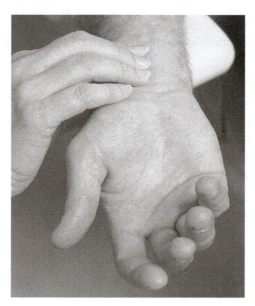

Figure 1-12 Measurement of the pulse at the radial artery

     iii. Women and children have a slightly elevated pulse.

     iv. A rapid pulse (tachycardia) may indicate nervousness or the presence of an infection, and a slow pulse (bradycardia) may indicate medication being taken or heart blockage.

     v. Locate the pulse with the pads of the first three fingers. Compress the artery to feel the pulse. Count the number of pulsations for a full minute. Note any irregularities.

  b. Respiration is defined as the inhalation and exhalation of air through the lungs.

     i. Sixteen to 20 breaths per minute is considered within normal limits.

     ii. Respiration is measured by observing the patient for one minute while patient is taking complete breaths.

     iii. Hyperventilation is the quick, short bursts of breaths being taken in, and hypoventilation is the sporadic bursts of breaths being taken in.

  c. Blood pressure is defined as the pressure of the blood in the circulatory system, often measured for diagnosis because it is related to the force and rate of the heartbeat and the diameter and elasticity of the arterial walls.

     i. Systole is the top reading and is the contraction of the chambers of the heart. Diastole is the bottom reading and is the phase of the heartbeat when the heart muscle relaxes and allows the chamber to fill with blood.

     ii. A baseline should be measured with a stethoscope and sphygmomanometer or an automatic blood pressure cuff and recorded in the patient chart. Readings at every appointment should be taken and recorded.

     iii. Normal blood pressure for an adult is **systolic** below 140 and **diastolic** below 90.

  d. Body temperature is defined as the level of heat produced and sustained by the body processes.

     i. Changes in body temperature can indicate disease.

     ii. A normal body temperature range for humans is between 98 and 99 degrees. A temperature of 98.6 degrees F is considered normal, but an elevated temperature can mean that the patient may be fighting an infection, usually bacterial in nature. A temperature below 97 degrees can mean hypothermia.

4. Recognize and describe abnormal findings in the head and neck.

  a. oral manifestations of systemic diseases

     i. bony structures providing support to teeth

     ii. alterations in musculature that affects chewing, swallowing, facial expressions, and talking

     iii. effects of diabetes

     iv. bacterial and fungal infections

     v. problems breathing, dryness in mouth and mucous membranes

     vi. pain or discomfort

     vii. discolorations, lesions, sores, rashes

  b. periodontal/diseases and conditions of the mucosa

     i. bleeding gums, loose teeth, inflamed gingiva, periodontal pockets, halitosis, pain, recession of gingiva discoloration

     ii. dental decay, trauma, sensitivity to heat and cold

  c. oral pathology that may be present

     i. inflammation

     ii. lesions

     iii. infection

     iv. congenital anomalies

     v. neoplasms

C. Charting

1. The Universal Numbering System is the most common form of dental charting found in the dental field (see Figures 1–9 and 1–13).

   a. Primary dentition begins on the upper right and ends on the lower right with teeth lettered A through T.

   b. Permanent dentition begins on the upper right and ends on the lower right with teeth numbered 1–32.

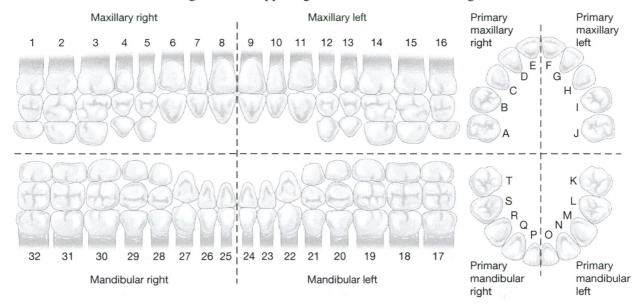

Figure 1-13 Universal Numbering System for both primary and deciduous dentition with identifying numbers and letters

   c. surfaces of the teeth (Figure 1-14)

      i. mesial: surface toward the midline
      ii. distal: surface away from the midline
      iii. occlusal: broad chewing surface of posterior teeth
      iv. incisal: biting surface of anterior teeth
      v. buccal: smooth surface of the posterior teeth that touches the cheek
      vi. facial: smooth surface of the anterior teeth that touches the lips
      vii. lingual: smooth surface of all teeth that touches the tongue

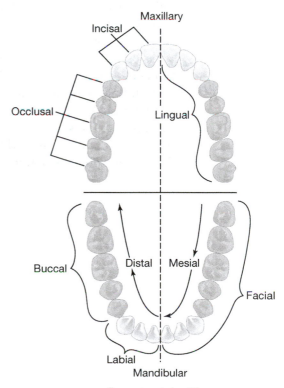

Permanent dentition

Figure 1-14 Surfaces of the teeth identified on the dental arches in a permanent dentition. Posterior teeth are shaded.

3. Accurately chart conditions in the patient's oral cavity (Figure 1-15)

   a. carious lesions

   b. existing conditions (usually charted using the color blue)

      i. restorations
      ii. missing teeth
      iii. impacted teeth
      iv. cysts and abnormalities
      v. other pathology of the hard tissues

   c. periodontal conditions

      i. periodontal pocket depth
      ii. tooth mobility
      iii. furcation involvement
      iv. gingival recession

   d. endodontic and periapical conditions

      i. pulpal disease: pulpitis, necrosis
      ii. periapical disease: periodontitis, abscess

   f. Charting must be accurate and becomes a part of the patient's legal dental history. Charting methods include:

      i. universal signs and symbols used to notate existing conditions or treatment to be completed in the chart.
      ii. blue pencil denotes existing treatment, while red pencil denotes treatment that needs to be completed.
      iii. Treatment notes should be in black ink. If there is a mistake, the mistake should be marked out with one single line, correct information noted below, and initialed by the person who entered the note. Some offices that use a computer will document treatment and administrative notes in different colors.
      iv. Notes on the computer should never be deleted, as most software programs have a feature that allows the recovery of deleted notes to prevent offices from altering notes in the event of a lawsuit. Enter new notes and indicate they are a correction and reference the correction by date.
      v. Being able to record accurate dental charting is both a legal as well as clinical necessity. While this information is useful in diagnosing and completing treatment, it is also mandatory in the event that your office is held liable for any results that may arise out of treatment. Accurate charting and documentation is a very important function of the dental assistant.

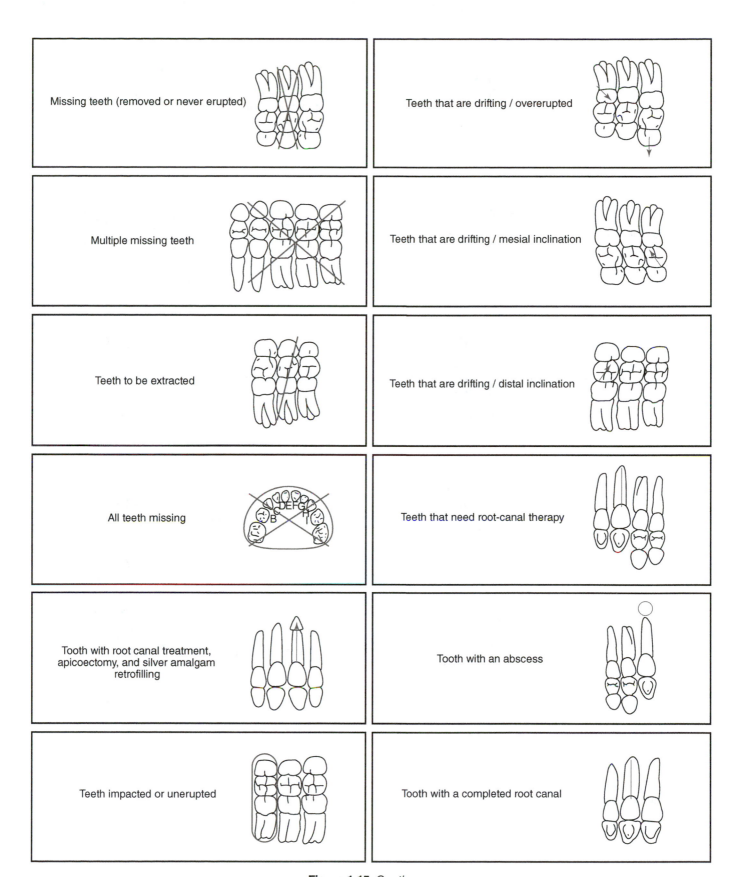

Missing teeth (removed or never erupted)

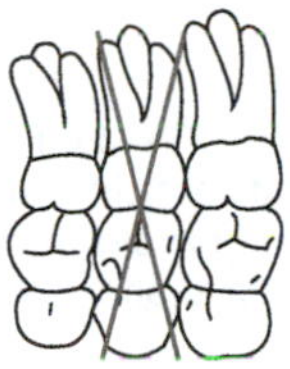

Teeth that are drifting / overerupted

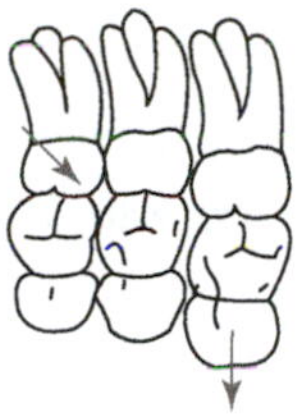

Multiple missing teeth

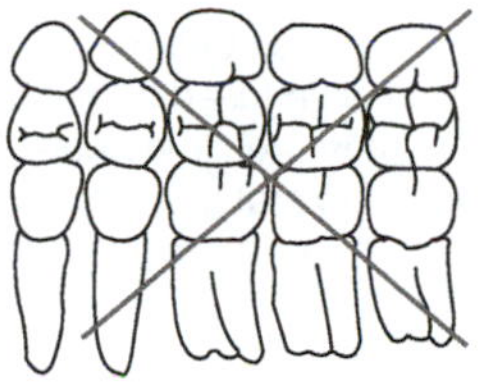

Teeth that are drifting / mesial inclination

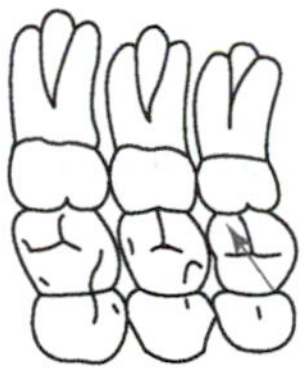

Teeth to be extracted

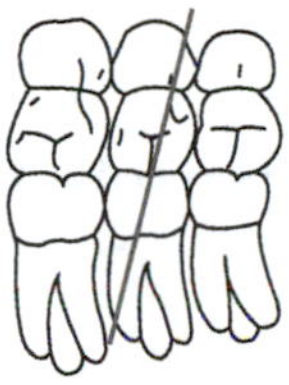

Teeth that are drifting / distal inclination

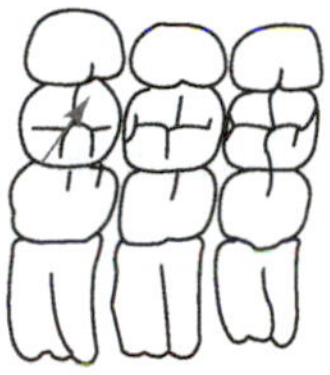

All teeth missing

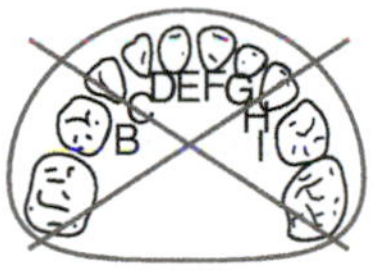

Teeth that need root-canal therapy

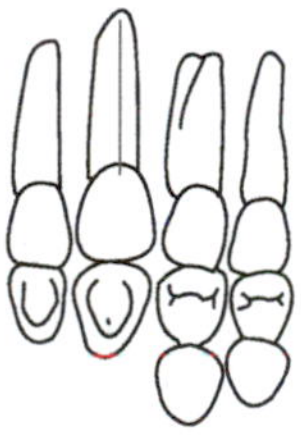

Tooth with root canal treatment, apicoectomy, and silver amalgam retrofilling

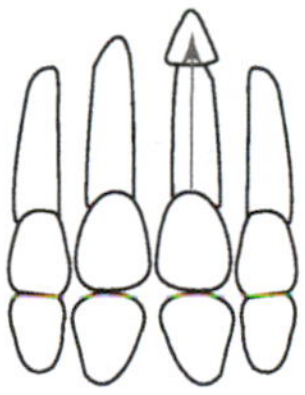

Tooth with an abscess

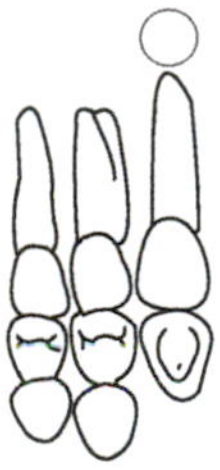

Teeth impacted or unerupted

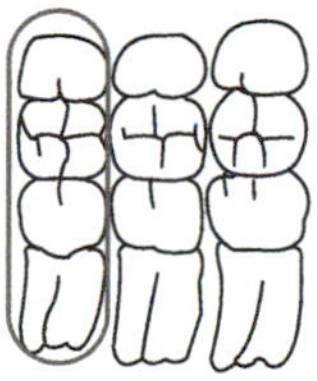

Tooth with a completed root canal

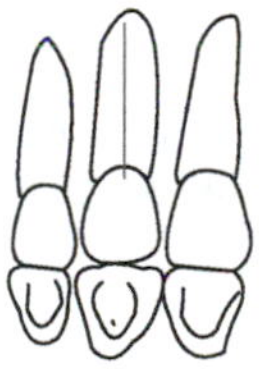

Figure 1-15 *Continues*

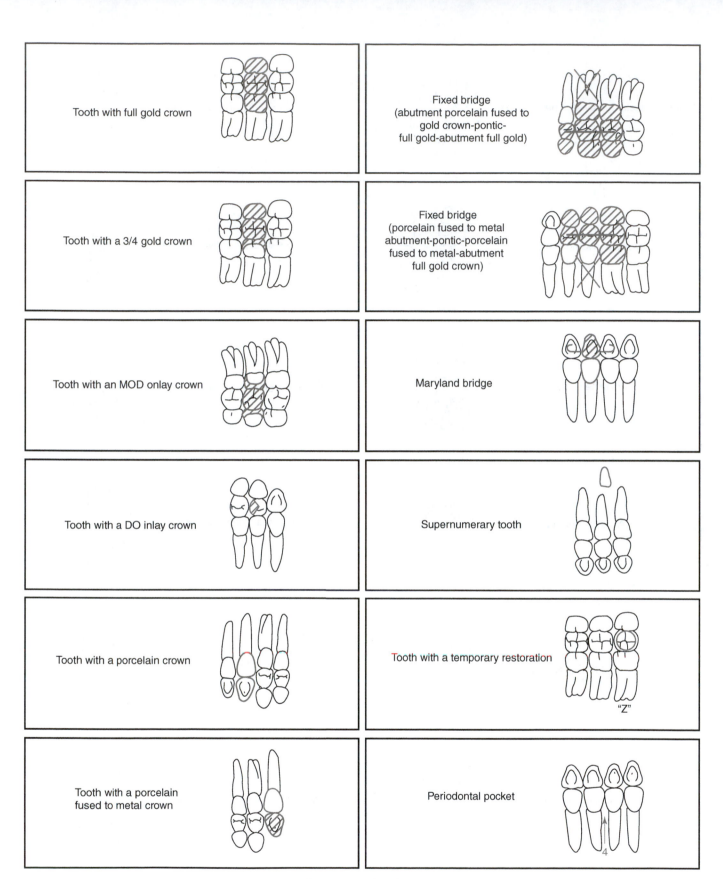

Tooth with full gold crown

Fixed bridge
(abutment porcelain fused to
gold crown-pontic-
full gold-abutment full gold)

Tooth with a 3/4 gold crown

Fixed bridge
(porcelain fused to metal
abutment-pontic-porcelain
fused to metal-abutment
full gold crown)

Tooth with an MOD onlay crown

Maryland bridge

Tooth with a DO inlay crown

Supernumerary tooth

Tooth with a porcelain crown

Tooth with a temporary restoration

"Z"

Tooth with a porcelain
fused to metal crown

Periodontal pocket

4

Figure 1-15 *Continues*

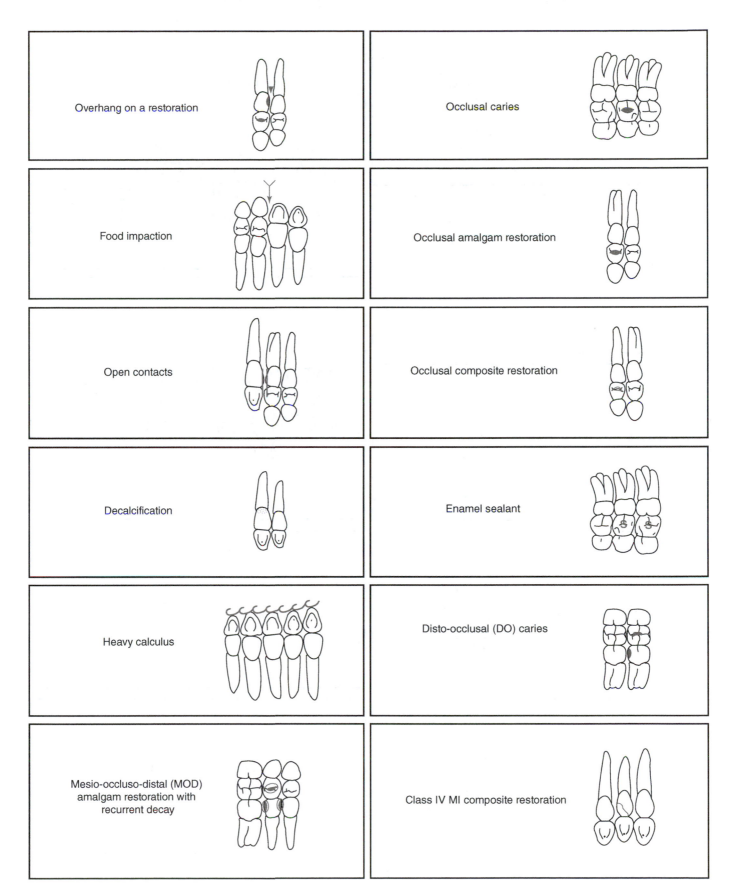

Overhang on a restoration	Occlusal caries
Food impaction	Occlusal amalgam restoration
Open contacts	Occlusal composite restoration
Decalcification	Enamel sealant
Heavy calculus	Disto-occlusal (DO) caries
Mesio-occluso-distal (MOD) amalgam restoration with recurrent decay	Class IV MI composite restoration

Figure 1-15 *Continues*

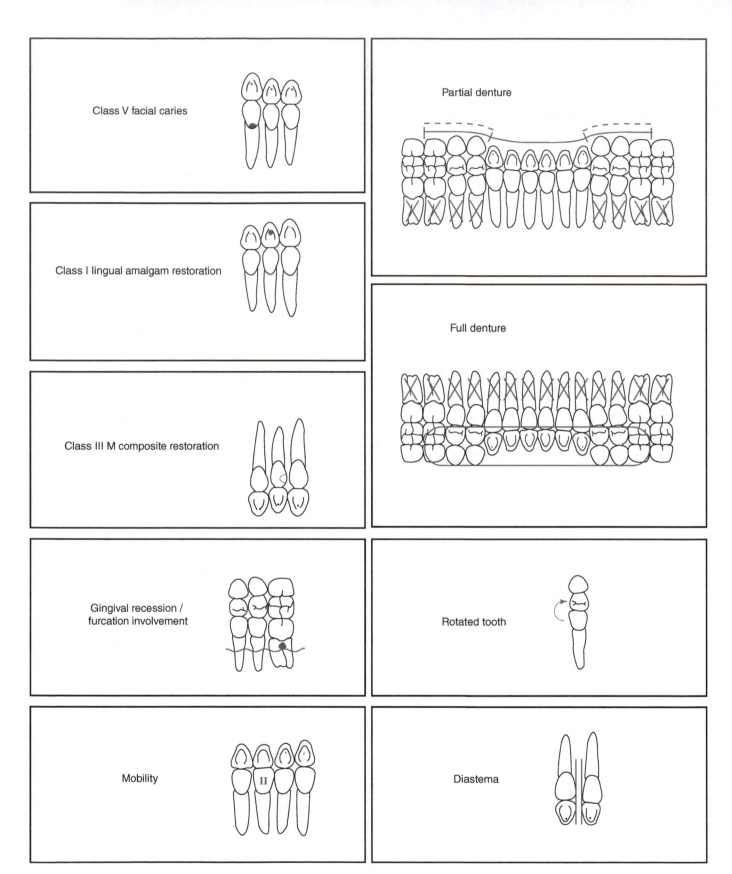

Class V facial caries

Class I lingual amalgam restoration

Class III M composite restoration

Gingival recession / furcation involvement

Mobility

Partial denture

Full denture

Rotated tooth

Diastema

Figure 1-15 *Continues*

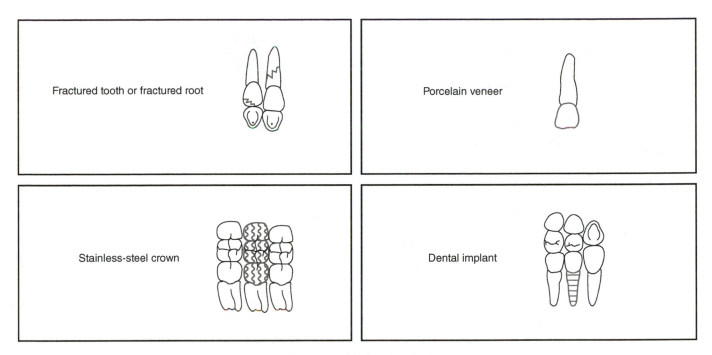

Figure 1-15 Charting symbols

D. Diagnostic Aids
    1. methods of diagnostic data collection
        a. study models
            i. bite mechanics/alignment
            ii. assessment and planning of orthodontic or cosmetic treatments
        b. radiographs
            i. evaluation and diagnosis of diseases of bony structures
            ii. evaluation and diagnosis of diseases of tooth structures
        c. pulp testing
            i. evaluation of vital and nonvital pulp
        d. extra- and intraoral photographs
            i. assessment and planning of orthodontic or cosmetic treatments
    2. Take and pour impressions for study models
E. Treatment Documentation
    1. Record treatment and medications prescribed by the dental office in the patient's chart
        a. understand parts of a prescription (Figure 1-16)
    2. Record recommended treatment and patient's acceptance or refusal of recommended treatment
        a. Record patient's acknowledgement of Health Insurance Portability and Accountability Act (HIPAA)
        b. Record any acceptance of patient information in regard to dental materials that may be used in the course of treatment
        c. Document and record patient refusal of any recommended treatment
    3. Record patient's compliance

Parts of a Prescription

1. The heading includes the dentist's name, address, telephone number, and registration number.

2. The superscription includes the patient's name, address, and the date on which the prescription is written.

3. The *subscription* that includes the symbol Rx ("take thou").

4. The *inscription* that states the names and quantities of ingredients to be included in the medication.

5. The *subscription* that gives directions to the pharmacist for filling the prescription.

6. The *signature* (Sig) that gives the directions for the patient.

7. The dentist's signature blanks. Where signed, indicates if a generic substitute is allowed or if the medication is to be dispensed as written.

8. REPETATUR 0 1 2 3 p.r.n. This is where the dentist indicates whether or not the prescription can be refilled.

9. ☐ LABEL Direction to the pharmacist to label the medication appropriately.

[1]
[2]
[3]
[4]
[5]
[6]
[7]
[8]
[9]

---

[1] L&K LEWIS & KING, DDS
2501 CENTER STREET
NORTHBOROUGH, OH 12345
CK 1424326

[2] Name___Juanita Hansen___

Address ___143 Gregory Lane, Apt. 43___ Date ___4/7/--___

[3] Rx

[4] Amoxicillin   500 mg

[5] Disp. #40

[6] Sig   1 cap qid x 10 days

[7] Generic Substitution Allowed ___Susan Lewis___
                                                    D.D.S.

Dispense As Written _____

[8] REPETATUR 0 1 2 3 p.r.n.   D.D.S.

[9] ☐ LABEL

Figure 1-16 Prescription with parts identified: (1) heading; (2) superscription; (3) Rx symbol; (4) inscription; (5) subscription; (6) signature; (7) signature for generic; (8) refills; and (9) labeling

Important Objectives to Know

1. Thoroughly understand basic dental anatomy and physiology.
2. Demonstrate general knowledge of what happens during the preliminary examination and the role of the dental assistant in the examination.
3. Demonstrate and interpret universal dental charting.
4. Explain how diagnostic data are collected.
5. Demonstrate the correct method of treatment recording.
6. Demonstrate how to take, record, and interpret vital signs.

Study Checklist

1. Review terminology as it relates to head and neck anatomy and physiology.
2. Review charting symbols and their meaning.
3. Understand why it is necessary to collect patient data and conduct the preliminary examination.
4. Review and be able to interpret patient vital signs and their ranges.

Section I:
Collection and Recording of Clinical Data –
Review Questions

Use the Answer Sheet found in Appendix A.

1. The frenum is
   a. a narrow band of tissue that connects two structures.
   b. a mucous membrane that lines the entire oral cavity.
   c. the corner of the mouth where the lips join.
   d. the retromolar area.

2. Bone that is more dense and forms the outer shell of bony structures is called:
   a. compact.
   b. cancellous.
   c. spongy.
   d. osseous.

3. There are _____ bones in the face.
   a. 14
   b. 18
   c. 22
   d. 28

4. The largest of the salivary glands is
   a. submandibular.
   b. parotid.
   c. sublingual.
   d. located under the jaw.

5. There are _____ bones in the cranium.
   a. 8
   b. 12
   c. 15
   d. 22

6. The salivary glands that lie on the floor of the mouth are the
   a. submandibular.
   b. parotid.
   c. sublingual.
   d. largest.

7. The salivary glands that lie on either side of the tongue are called
   a. submandibular.
   b. parotid.
   c. sublingual.
   d. Wharton's.

8. The duct that comes off the parotid gland is called
   a. Wharton's duct.
   b. Stensen's duct.
   c. ducts of Rivinus.
   d. submandibular.

9. Spongy bone is also known as
   a. cortical bone.
   b. cancellous bone.
   c. crustiform bone.
   d. diatomaceous.

10. Muscle origin is the place where the
    a. muscle ends.
    b. muscle begins.
    c. muscle inserts.
    d. muscle is at its strongest.

11. The duct that comes off of the sublingual gland is called
    a. Wharton's duct.
    b. Stensen's duct.
    c. ducts of Rivinus.
    d. the sublingual duct.

12. The muscle that closes and puckers the lips is known as the
    a. mentalis.
    b. orbicularis oris.
    c. orbicularis oculi.
    d. buccinators.

13. The muscle that compresses the cheeks against the teeth and retracts the angle of the mouth is known as the
    a. frontalis muscle.
    b. orbicularis oris muscle.
    c. buccinator muscle.
    d. zygomatic minor muscle.

14. The strongest muscle of the jaw used for chewing is known as the
    a. masseter muscle.
    b. buccinator muscle.
    c. mentalis muscle.
    d. zygomatic minor muscle.

15. After taking the temperature on a patient, the "dental assistant notes the temperature as being 99.8 degrees F. This may indicate which of the following situations?
    a. hypothermia
    b. blood loss
    c. illness such as a headache or intestinal upset
    d. bacterial infection

16. During the intraoral examination, the dentist tells you there is an existing crown on tooth #30. How would you make the notation on the patient chart?
    a. in red on the lower right second molar
    b. in blue on the lower left first bicuspid
    c. in red on the upper right first molar
    d. in blue on the lower right second molar

17. After performing a medical history review, the patient tells you that she is allergic to penicillin. How would you notate this in the patient chart?
    a. in the treatment notes in red pencil
    b. on the cover of the chart in red pen
    c. in the insurance notes in red pen
    d. on the registration page of the chart in green pen

18. This muscle raises and wrinkles the skin of the chin and pushes up the lower lip.
    a. buccinator
    b. mentalis
    c. orbicularis oris
    d. zygomatic minor

19. The portion of the tooth covered with enamel is known as the
    a. anatomic crown.
    b. clinical crown.
    c. coronal crown.
    d. cortical crown.

20. The substance that covers the root of the tooth is called
    a. periodontal ligament.
    b. cementum.
    c. dentin.
    d. Sharpey's fibers.

21. The portion of the tooth that is visible in the mouth is called the
    a. anatomical crown.
    b. anatomical root.
    c. clinical crown.
    d. clinical root.

22. Which of these is a muscle of mastication?
    a. mentalis
    b. masseter
    c. zygomatic minor
    d. orbicularis oris

23. The enamel of the tooth
    a. is the material that covers the anatomical crown.
    b. is the material that covers the root of the tooth.
    c. can be considered the bulk of the tooth.
    d. is part of the root of the tooth.

24. The pulp can best be described as
    a. covering the root of the tooth.
    b. consisting of tissue that surrounds and supports the teeth.
    c. nourishes and protects the tooth.
    d. the hardest substance in the body.

25. It can be stated that the occlusal surface of the tooth is
    a. the anterior chewing surface of the dentition.
    b. located on the bicuspids only.
    c. the broad, flat chewing surface of the posterior teeth.
    d. restored using a class V restoration.

26. There are _____ teeth in the primary dentition.
    a. 20
    b. 24
    c. 30
    d. 32

Complete the following questions regarding dental charting (Figure 1-17).

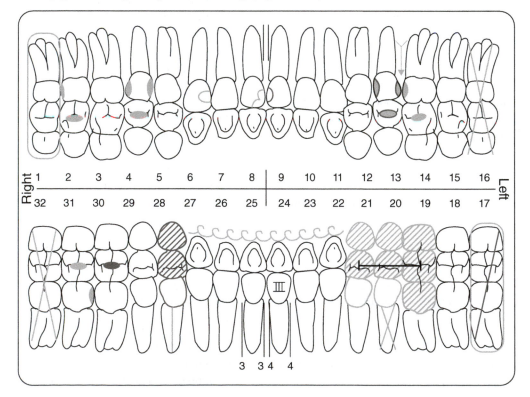

Figure 1-17 Charting exercise

27. Tooth #7 is
    a. missing.
    b. impacted.
    c. abscessed.
    d. drifting mesially.

28. Tooth #30 has a/an
    a. root canal.
    b. occlusal restoration.
    c. incisal restoration.
    d. gold crown

29. Tooth #28 has a
    a. ¾ gold crown.
    b. ¾ porcelain crown.
    c. ¾ composite crown.
    d. root canal.

30. Tooth # 8 needs a
    a. mesio-incisal composite.
    b. disto-incisal composite.
    c. composite crown.
    d. mesio-occlusal composite.

31. Tooth #13 needs a
    a. class I restoration.
    b. class II restoration.
    c. class V restoration.
    d. class VI restoration.

32. Tooth #32
    a. is missing.
    b. needs to be extracted.
    c. is impacted.
    d. has decay present.

33. Teeth #24 and #25
    a. have mobility.
    b. have furcation involved periodontal disease.
    c. have periodontal pocketing.
    d. need to be extracted.

34. While transcribing treatment information into a chart, you realize you have made a mistake. The best way to notate this is by doing which of the following?
    a. Erase it and write in the correct information.
    b. White it out and write in the correct information.
    c. Cross the inaccuracy out with a single straight line, write in the correct information below, and then initial next to it.
    d. Do nothing; it is illegal to alter the chart in any way.

35. All existing restorations are charted in
    a. red.
    b. blue.
    c. green.
    d. black.

36. Restorative work that needs to be done is
    a. charted in blue.
    b. charted in green.
    c. charted in red.
    d. not charted at all.

37. The _____ surface refers to the surface that is toward the midline.
    a. distal
    b. mesial
    c. median
    d. sagittal

38. The sharp, biting edge of the anterior teeth is referred to as
    a. facial.
    b. occlusal.
    c. incisal.
    d. buccal.

39. During an oral examination, the assistant is responsible for all of the following EXCEPT
    a. assisting the patient in completing the medical and dental history.
    b. recording all of the dentist's findings.
    c. recommending needed treatment.
    d. assisting in the preparation of the patient and room for treatment.

40. A normal pulse is between _____ beats per minute.
    a. 45 and 60
    b. 60 and 100
    c. 100 and 150
    d. 150 and 200

41. In the dental field, the most common area where the pulse is taken on adults is the
    a. carotid artery.
    b. radial artery.
    c. brachial artery.
    d. femoral artery.

42. Masticatory mucosa covers
    a. the root of the tooth.
    b. the areas subject to stress.
    c. the tongue.
    d. the inside of the cheek.

43. The largest muscle of mastication is referred to as
    a. temporalis.
    b. masseter.
    c. buccinator.
    d. orbicularis oris.

44. There are no _____ in the primary dentition.
    a. first molars, bicuspids
    b. bicuspids, third molars
    c. lateral incisors, bicuspids
    d. cuspids, third molars

45. The single bone that forms the inferior portion of the nasal septum is referred to as
    a. lacrimal bone.
    b. inferior nasal conchae.
    c. vomer.
    d. nasal bone.

46. Which blood vessel branches to form the right common carotid artery?
    a. brachiocephalic artery
    b. internal carotid artery
    c. external carotid artery
    d. vertebral artery

47. The left common carotid artery divides to form which artery?
    a. external and internal carotid artery
    b. external and internal subclavian artery
    c. internal jugular
    d. external jugular

48. The internal jugular vein drains via the cranium from which structures?
    a. neck area and left arm
    b. parotid glands
    c. neck and right arm
    d. brain and neck

49. External jugular veins drain from which structures?
    a. parotid glands, facial muscles, and scalp
    b. brain and neck
    c. neck and left arm
    d. superior vena cava

50. The broad chewing surface of a posterior molar is referred to as
    a. incisal.
    b. buccal.
    c. distal.
    d. occlusal.

51. How many teeth are found in the adult permanent dentition?
    a. 24
    b. 28
    c. 30
    d. 32

52. Name the bone that comprises the cheek.
    a. hyoid
    b. zygomatic
    c. occipital
    d. maxilla

53. Name the pendulous attachment of tissue that hangs in the back of the throat.
    a. lingual frenum
    b. uvula
    c. rugae
    d. epiglottis

54. The mucosa that covers the area subject to stress such as gingival tissue and the hard palate are referred to what mucosa?
    a. masticatory mucosa
    b. specialized mucosa
    c. lining mucosa
    d. buccal mucosa

55. Which cranial bone forms the forehead, frontal sinuses, and upper orbits of the eye?
    a. ethmoid
    b. frontal
    c. sphenoid
    d. mandible

56. The distal portion of the tooth refers to which surface?
    a. the surface toward the midline
    b. the surface away from the midline
    c. the chewing surface
    d. the surface closest to the gingival

57. The surface of the posterior teeth that touches the cheek is referred to as which surface?
    a. distal
    b. facial
    c. buccal
    d. incisal

58. Part of taking the preliminary medical history includes which activity?
    a. establishing the purpose of the patient's visit
    b. assessment of patient's physical condition
    c. record patient's chief complaint
    d. any of the above

59. When a tooth is circled in red on a patient chart, this could generally mean what about the tooth?
    a. The tooth has a porcelain crown.
    b. The tooth is impacted.
    c. The tooth needs to be extracted.
    d. The tooth is missing.

60. When a tooth has a solid red line going through the roots, this could generally mean what about the tooth?
    a. It is a full gold crown.
    b. It is in need of endodontic treatment.
    c. It is unerupted.
    d. It is impacted.

61. When taking a recording of blood pressure and you get a reading of 130/72, which number is referred to as the diastolic?
    a. 130
    b. 72
    c. 200
    d. 54

62. When a taking a patient's temperature, a normal reading is considered to be what?
    a. 97.6 degrees F
    b. 98.6 degrees F
    c. 98.4 degrees F
    d. 99.6 degrees F

63. All existing restorations, using the Universal Charting System, are charted with what color pencil?
    a. red
    b. blue
    c. green
    d. black

64. Teeth that are charted to be extracted, using the Universal Charting system, are marked using which symbol?
   a. a red "X" through the tooth
   b. a red diagonal line through the entire tooth
   c. a red circle around the tooth
   d. a red circle around the crown only

65. Teeth that have an abscess, using the Universal Charting system, are marked using which symbol?
   a. an "X" over the apex
   b. the entire tooth circled in red
   c. the entire root circled in red
   d. the apex of the tooth circled in red

66. How do teeth that have been sealed appear when using the Universal Charting system?
   a. a blue "S" on the occlusal surface
   b. a blue "S" on the facial surface
   c. a blue "S" on the lingual surface
   d. none of the above

67. When charting restorations, a PFM is the abbreviation for which occurrence?
   a. patient faints momentarily
   b. porcelain fused to metal crown
   c. porcelain filling on mesial surface
   d. porcelain finished material

68. Vitals can be considered all of the following except which choice?
   a. respiration
   b. heart rate or pulse
   c. weight
   d. blood pressure

69. An intraoral examination consists of all of the following except which choice?
   a. the dentist examining the patient's tonsils
   b. the dentist examining the patient's tongue
   c. the dentist examining facial symmetry
   d. the assistant observing and recording existing restorations

70. When charting, the universal meaning for FGC is commonly noted as being what?
   a. facial gold classification
   b. fine-grade composite
   c. full gold crown
   d. first gold crown

71. The sharp, biting edge of the anterior teeth is referred to as which surface?
   a. facial
   b. buccal
   c. mesial
   d. incisal

72. Which tooth system uses a numbering system of 1–32 for permanent teeth and lettering from A–T?
   a. Universal Numbering System
   b. Palmer notation
   c. ADA system
   d. Classic Classification

73. If a mistake is made in the computer chart documentation, the best course of action is to do which of the following?
   a. Remove the entire notation and insert a new one with the correct information.
   b. Note that there is an error in the note below the original entry and type in your initial.
   c. Make an entry on the day you notice the mistake, note the mistake and date of mistake and type the correct information in and include your name at the end.
   d. Tell the dentist and let him make the correction.

Section I:
Collection and Recording of Clinical Data –
Answers and Rationales

1. The frenum is

   a. a narrow band of tissue that connects two structures.

2. Bone that is more dense and forms the outer shell of bony structures is called

   a. compact.

3. There are _____ bones in the face.

   a. 14

4. The largest of the salivary glands are

   b. parotid.

5. There are ____ bones in the cranium.

   a. 8

6. The salivary glands that lie on the floor of the mouth are the

   c. sublingual.

7. The salivary glands that lie on either side of the tongue are called

   c. sublingual.

8. The duct that comes off the parotid gland is called

   b. Stensen's duct.

9. Spongy bone is also known as

   b. cancellous bone.

10. Muscle origin is the place where the

    b. muscle begins.

11. The duct that comes off of the sublingual gland is called

    a. Wharton's duct.

12. The muscle that closes and puckers the lips and is known as the

    b. orbicularis oris.

13. The muscle that compresses the cheeks against the teeth and retracts the angle of the mouth is known as the

    c. buccinator muscle.

14. The strongest muscle of the jaw used for chewing is known as the

    a. masseter muscle.

15. After taking the temperature on a patient, the dental assistant notes the temperature as being 99.8 degrees F. This may indicate which of the following situations?

    d. bacterial infection – Bacterial infections are accompanied by fever. Viral infections do not usually present with fever.

16. During the intraoral examination, the dentist tells you there is an existing crown on tooth #30. How would you make the notation on the patient chart?

    d. in blue on the lower right first molar

17. After performing a medical history review, the patient tells you that she is allergic to penicillin. How would you notate this in the patient chart?

    b. on the cover of the chart in red pen – Oftentimes if the office is paperless and notes are kept in the computer, this would present on a pop-up men. If it is neither in red pen on the front of a paper chart or is noted in the computer the patient is asked to verify allergy and the assistant can make the notation.

18. This muscle raises and wrinkles the skin of the chin and pushes up the lower lip.

    b. mentalis

19. The portion of the tooth covered with enamel is known as the

    b. clinical crown – This is the entire tooth, including the crown that is below the gingival crest.

20. The substance that covers the root of the tooth is called

    b. cementum.

21. The portion of the tooth that is visible in the mouth is called the

    c. clinical crown.

22. Which of these is a muscle of mastication?

    b. masseter

23. The enamel of the tooth

    a. is the material that covers the anatomical crown.

24. The pulp can best be described as

    c. nourishes and protects the tooth.

25. It can be stated that the occlusal surface of the tooth is

    c. the broad, flat chewing surface of the posterior teeth.

26. There are _____ teeth in the primary dentition.

    a. 20 – These teeth are also sometimes referred to as deciduous.

27. Tooth #17 is

    b. impacted.

28. Tooth #30 has an

    b. occlusal restoration.

29. Tooth #28 has a

　　a. ¾ gold crown.

30. Tooth #8 needs a

　　a. mesio-incisal composite.

31. Tooth #13 needs a

　　b. class II restoration.

32. Tooth #32

　　a. is missing.

33. Teeth #24 and #25

　　c. have periodontal pocketing – Periodontal pocket readings are measured using a periodontal probe, and the number, which can range from 1 mm to 10mm, is noted on the chart.

34. While transcribing treatment information into a chart, you realize you have made a mistake. The best way to notate this is by doing which of the following?

　　c. Cross the inaccuracy out with a single straight line, write in the correct information below, and then initial next to it. You should never erase or use Whiteout, as the chart is a legal document, and if it ever needs to be entered in as evidence and there is Whiteout or it appears that some of the notes have been altered, it will appear that the office is trying to cover up a mistake.

35. All existing restorations are charted in

　　b. blue.

36. Restorative work that is diagnosed is

　　c. charted in red.

37. The _____ surface refers to the surface that is toward the midline.

　　b. mesial

38. The sharp, biting edge of the anterior teeth is referred to as

　　c. incisal.

39. During an oral examination, the assistant is responsible for all of the following EXCEPT

　　c. recommending needed treatment.

40. A normal pulse is between _____ beats per minute.

　　b. 60 and 100

41. In the dental field, the most common area where the pulse is taken on adults is the

　　b. radial artery.

42. Masticatory mucosa covers

　　b. the areas subject to stress such as the tongue.

43. The largest muscle of mastication is referred to as

　　b. masseter.

44. There are no _____ in the primary dentition.

　　b. bicuspids, third molars – These teeth appear as part of the permanent dentition.

45. The single bone that forms the inferior portion of the nasal septum is referred to as

　　c. vomer.

46. Which blood vessel branches to form the right common carotid artery?

　　a. brachiocephalic trunk

47. The left common carotid artery divides to form which artery?

　　a. external and internal carotid artery

48. The internal jugular vein drains via the cranium from which structures?

　　d. brain and neck

49. External jugular veins drain which structures?

　　a. parotid glands, facial muscles, and scalp

50. The broad chewing surface of a posterior molar is referred to as

　　a. occlusal.

51. How many teeth are found in the adult permanent dentition?

　　d. 32

52. Name the bone that comprises the cheek.

　　b. Zygomatic – this bone and its process form the arch of the cheekbone.

53. Name the pendulous attachment of tissue that hangs in the back of the throat.

　　b. Uvula – This is the tissue that is located at the back of the throat. It is not known what its purpose is, but it has been linked to snoring and sleep apnea.

54. The mucosa that covers the area subject to stress such as gingival tissue and the hard palate are referred to what mucosa?

　　a. Masticatory mucosa – These areas are able to withstand the forces of chewing and other stresses without tearing easily.

55. Which cranial bone forms the forehead, frontal sinuses, and upper orbits of the eye?

　　b. Frontal – The frontal bone is a single bone that is also known as the forehead.

56. The distal portion of the tooth refers to which surface?

　　b. the surface away from the midline – The surface away from the midline is referred to as the distal surface. These surfaces can be remembered by reminding yourself it's the surface heading toward the back of the mouth.

57. The surface of the posterior teeth that touches the cheek is referred to as which surface?

   c. **buccal – The buccal surface is the surface where the posterior teeth touch the cheek. For the anterior teeth, this surface is referred to as facial.**

58. Part of taking the preliminary medical history includes which activity?

   d. **any of the above – Establishing the purpose of the visit, assessment of the patient and their physical condition, and recording their chief complaint are all part of the preliminary medical history.**

59. When a tooth is circled in red on a patient chart, this could generally mean what about the tooth?

   b. **The tooth is impacted.**

60. When a tooth has a solid red line going through the roots, this could generally mean what about the tooth?

   b. **It is in need of endodontic treatment.**

61. When taking a recording of blood pressure and you get a reading of 130/72, which number is referred to as the diastolic?

   b. **72 – Diastolic is always the reading on the bottom.**

62. When a taking a patient's temperature, a normal reading is considered to be what?

   b. **98.6 degrees F – This is considered "normal." Some patients can have a degree differential either way higher or lower and still be considered normal, for them.**

63. All existing restorations, using the Universal Charting System, are charted with what color pencil?

   b. **blue**

64. Teeth that are charted to be extracted, using the Universal Charting system, are marked using which symbol?

   a. **a red "X" through the tooth**

65. Teeth that have an abscess, using the Universal Charting system, are marked using which symbol?

   d. **the apex of the tooth circled in red – Only the apex of the root that is diseased is circled in red.**

66. How do teeth that have been sealed appear when using the Universal Charting system?

   a. **a blue "S" on the occlusal surface – Only posterior teeth are routinely sealed.**

67. When charting restorations, a PFM is the abbreviation for which occurrence?

   b. **porcelain fused to metal crown**

68. Vitals can be considered all of the following except which choice?

   c. **weight – This is not considered part of the collection of vitals in the dental office.**

69. An intraoral examination consists of all of the following except which choice?

   c. **the dentist examining facial symmetry – This is not considered part of an intraoral examination. This is the only observation that is noted extraorally.**

70. When charting, the universal meaning for FGC is commonly noted as being what?

   c. **full gold crown**

71. The sharp, biting edge of the anterior teeth is referred to as which surface?

   d. **incisal – The incisal surface occurs on the anterior teeth.**

72. Which tooth system uses a numbering system of 1–32 for permanent teeth and lettering from A–T?

   a. **Universal Numbering System**

73. If a mistake is made in chart documentation, on the computer the best course of action it do which of the following?

   c. **Make an entry on the day you notice the mistake, note the mistake and date of mistake and type the correct information in and include your name at the end.**

Section II: Chairside Dental Procedures

This section of the General Chairside portion of the Certified Dental Assisting Examination consists of 45% or 54 questions of the 120 multiple-choice items. The questions related to this section of the General Chairside Dental Assisting Examination are based upon your knowledge of the following:

- Four-handed dentistry techniques
- Selection and preparation of armamentarium
- Performing or assisting with intraoral procedures
- Patient-management techniques

Key Terms

armamentarium – all materials and instruments needed to complete a dental procedure
four-handed dentistry – system in which the dentist and dental assistant work together at the dental chair
nitrous oxide – odor-free gas derived from nitrogen and oxygen; used as a sedative before anesthesia
static zone – the activity zone where rear delivery systems are located along with dental instruments and equipment used at the dental chair
transfer zone – the area below the patient's nose where instruments and materials are passed and received

Quick Review Outline

A. The dental assistant should be familiar with the following **four-handed dentistry** techniques

1. When preparing the treatment room for the patient, ideally, the assistant should have the treatment room completely set up with all of the materials and instruments that will be needed for the procedure. The assistant should not have to leave the operator's side to retrieve any items unless they are unusual items that would not ordinarily be used. The treatment room must be set up following all infection-control standards.

2. When preparing the treatment trays with **armamentarium**, they are placed in the sequence of use and delivery position. Instruments are arranged in order of use. This facilitates the procedure and keeps everything organized for both operator and assistant.

3. The assistant should be able to seat and prepare the patient and position and adjust equipment or instruments needed for the appointment.

   a. Patients are seated in a subsupine position during treatment. This creates a situation in which the patient's head is slightly below their heart. This places the patient's head directly in the operator's lap area, which provides for maximum access to the oral cavity.

4. The assistant should be familiar with implementing four-handed dentistry concepts during treatment procedures. This will facilitate efficiency between the operator and the assistant. This concept reduces the need for the operator to look away from the patient or become distracted with other responsibilities but instead provides the opportunity for the operator to dedicate their full attention to the patient while having the assistant provide the materials chairside. The assistant should focus on the following:

   a. Assume correct positions for procedures. The assistant should sit approximately six inches higher than the operator.

   b. For the right-handed operator, the assistant should be seated in the two to four o'clock position and the operator at the seven to twelve o'clock position (Figure 1-18A).

   c. For the left-handed operator, the dental assistant should be seated at the eight to ten o'clock position while the operator is seated at the twelve to five o'clock position (Figure 1-18B).

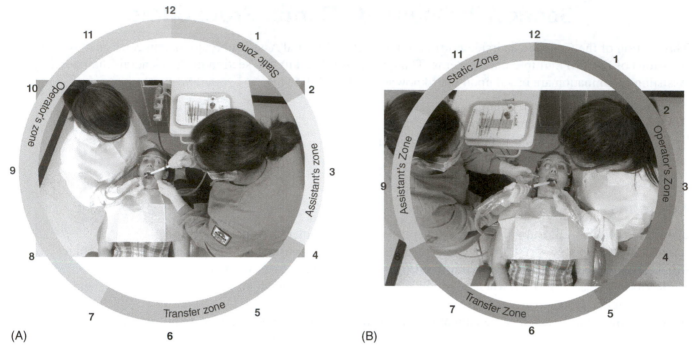

Figure 1-18 (A) Activity zones for a right-handed operator, with the assistant on the left. (B) Activity zones for a left-handed operator, with the assistant on the right.

   c. The **static zone** is the zone in which instruments and materials are passed during four-handed dentistry. For the right-handed operator, the static zone is between twelve and two o'clock. For the left-handed operator, it is between ten and twelve o'clock.

   d. The **transfer zone** is the area in which instruments are passed between the operator and the assistant. For the right-handed operator, this is between four and seven o'clock, and for the left-handed operator, it is between five and eight o'clock.

   e. Balance and posture for the dental assistant are important to reduce fatigue and place you in the best position to pass and receive instruments and materials.

      i. The assistant must be able to see and have access to the oral cavity.

      ii. The assistant must be able to pass instruments, retract tissues, evacuate fluids, and maintain a clear field at all time for the operator.

     iii. The assistant must be able to keep an erect posture, use the support arm to support the upper body, and be seated in the middle of the assistant chair seat.

     iv. Instruments and bracket table should be within easy reach of the assistant.

     v. Eliminating unnecessary movements by both the assistant and the operator is one of the goals of efficient assisting. This saves time and effort and speeds the time required for procedures.

   f. Successful instrument transfer is based on a set of principles that require organization and planning.

   g. Knowing the treatment plan and the materials needed to deliver that treatment should be planned well in advance.

   h. Know how to execute the various procedures and the development of a standardized routine for each procedure.

   i. Instrument grasps (Figure 1-19 A–D]

      i. The pen grasp resembles the position commonly used to hold a pen or pencil and is widely used for most operative instruments.

      ii. The modified pen grasp is similar to the pen grasp except the operator uses the pad of the middle finger on the handle of the instrument.

     iii. The palm grasp is used for bulky instruments. It is commonly used for surgical forceps, rubber damp clamp forceps, straight chisels and the air/water syringe.

     iv. The palm-thumb or thumb-to-nose grasp is used by the assistant for holding the high-velocity evacuator.

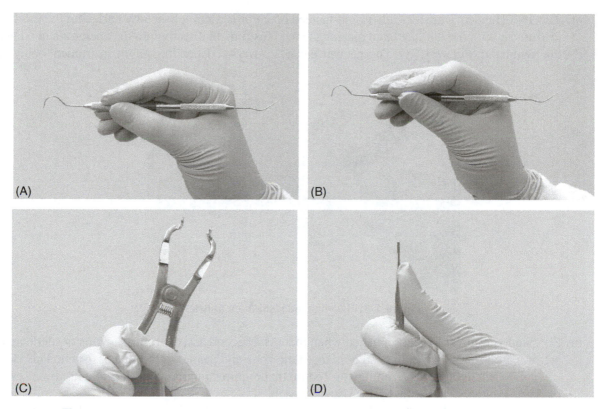

Figure 1-19 (A) Pen grasp. (B) Modified pen grasp. (C) Palm grasp. (D) Palm-thumb grasp.

j. The most common instrument transfers used today in dentistry are the single-handed, two-handed, and six-handed transfers. The assistant's hand is divided into two parts: the part that picks up the instrument and the part that delivers the instrument. We will address the fingers of the hand as the thumb, first, second, third, and fourth. Some assistants receive the used instrument with only the small finger. This could cause a problem for the assistant in keeping control of the instrument, and he/she may drop it. For safety purposes, the assistant should retrieve the instrument using two fingers.

   i. Single-Handed Transfer Technique (Right-handed operator). The single-handed transfer is used during most restorative procedures. This transfer requires that the assistant pass instruments with the thumb and first finger of the left hand and hold the oral evacuator tip and air/water syringe in the right hand. If the assistant is working with a left-handed operator, all the positions described here are reversed. Retrieving the instrument is accomplished by extending the third and fourth finger of the left hand, and as you receive the instrument with the third and fourth finger, you are using the first finger and thumb in the modified pen grasp; place the next instrument of use into the operator's hand (Figure 1-20).

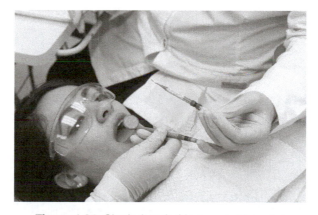

Figure 1-20 Single-handed instrument transfer

ii. The Two-Handed Transfer with a right-handed operator is accomplished by retrieving the used instrument with the left hand and placing the next instrument directly into the operator's hand using the right hand (Figure 1-21). This sequence can be reversed depending on the instrument being passed.

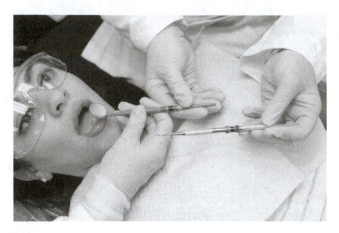

Figure 1-21 Two-handed instrument transfer

iii. Six-handed transfer is accomplished when there is a second assistant. Instruments or medicaments are prepared by the second assistant in the static zone and passed to the first assistant. This is most often used when there is a complex procedure that requires mixing materials that are time sensitive or there are items out of the first assistant's reach.

iv. Key item to remember is that all instruments must be passed under the patient's chin or over their chest and never over their face.

B. Selection and preparation of armamentarium – the assistant should be familiar with the following:

1. Selecting, preparing, and/or modifying impression trays for appropriate uses by using wax or by heating and manipulating the tray. If appropriate, adding wax to the periphery or using heat to manipulate plastic trays help to achieve an impression that captures all of the anatomical features required.

2. Selecting and preparing tray setups and all necessary armamentaria for general dentistry and dental emergency procedures is part of the assistant's responsibility. The operator has to be focused on the procedure and not preoccupied with whether the room is properly set up. This is the responsibility of the assistant.

a. Anesthetic tray (Figure 1-22)

i. Appropriate needle with recapping device
ii. Appropriate anesthesia
iii. Cotton-tip applicator
iv. Local topical anesthesia
v. Disposable items

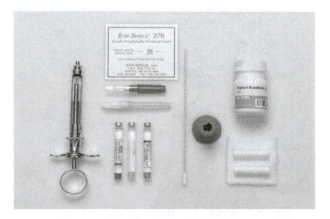

Figure 1-22 Tray setup for anesthesia

b. Amalgam restoration tray (Figure 1-23)

    i. Basic setup
    ii. Anesthetic setup
    iii. Appropriate burs
    iv. Bases, liners, or varnish
    v. Matrix band and retainer
    vi. Amalgam, amalgam carrier, and amalgam well
    vii. Condensers, burnishers, and carvers
    viii. Articulating paper and holder
    ix. Disposable items

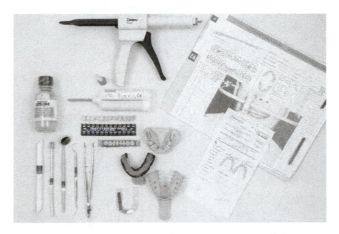

Figure 1-23 Tray setup for amalgam restoration

c. Composite restorations tray (Figure 1-24)

    i. Basic setup
    ii. Anesthetic setup
    iii. Appropriate burs
    iv. Composite materials including etch, primer, and bond
    v. Condensers, burnisher, carvers
    vii. Matrix band and retainer
    viii. Curing light
    ix. Disposable items

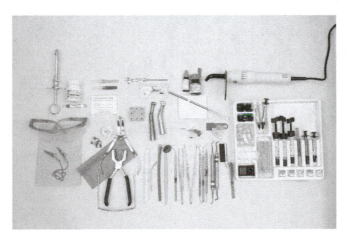

Figure 1-24 Tray setup for composite restoration

d. Crown and bridge preparation/cementation tray (Figure 1-25A and B)

    i. Basic setup

    ii. Anesthetic setup

    iii. Diamond burs and finishing stones

    iv. Gingival cord placement instrument and cord

    v. Impression materials and trays

    vi. Temporary cement, spatula, and mixing pad

    vii. Disposable items

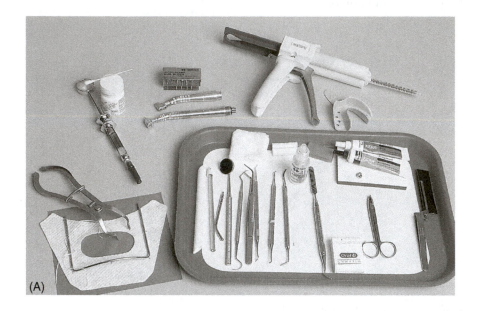

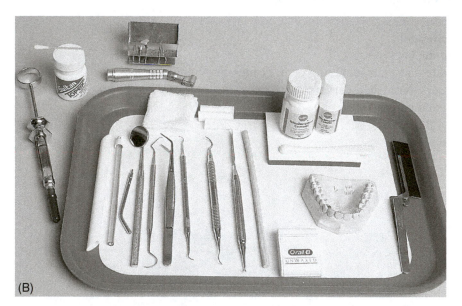

Figure 1-25 (A) Tray setup for crown and bridge preparation appointment. (B) Tray setup for crown and bridge cementation appointment.

e. Tooth desensitization

    i. Basic setup

    ii. Desensitizing solution

    iii. Brushes or applicators

    iv. Disposable items

f. Endodontic therapy tray (Figure 1-26A and B)

    i. Basic setup

    ii. Anesthetic setup

    iii. Files, broaches, and reamers

    iv. Medicaments

    v. Spreaders, pluggers, and explorers

    vi. Gutta percha, sealers, and canal filling materials

    vii. Disposable items

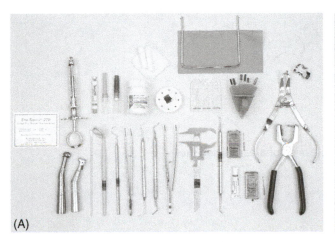
(A)

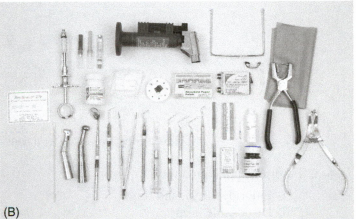
(B)

Figure 1-26 (A) Root canal treatment tray setup, opening appointment. (A) Mouth mirror. (B) Explorer. (C) Cotton pliers. (D) Endodontic explorer. (E) Endodontic spoon excavator. (F) Locking cotton pliers. (G) Cotton rolls/gauze sponge. (H) Bur block. (I) Anesthetic setup. (J) Dental dam set up. (K) High-speed handpiece. (L) Low-speed handpiece. (M) Millimeter ruler. (N) Paper points. (O) Barbed broach, assorted reamers and files, with stops in endodontic organizer. (P) Peeso reamers. (Q) Gates-Glidden drills. (R) Glick endodontic instrument. (S) Temporary filling material. (B) Root canal completion appointment tray setup. (A) Mouth mirror. (B) Endodontic explorer. (C) Locking cotton pliers. (D) Endodontic spoon excavator. (E) Irrigating syringe. (F) Burs. (G) High and low-speed handpieces. (H) Spreaders. (I) Pluggers. (J) Spatula. (K) Glick instrument. (L) Gates-Glidden drills. (M) Absorbent sterile paper points. (N) Lentulo spiral. (O) Gutta percha. (P) Root canal sealer. (Q) Heat source. (R) Rubber dam setup. (S) Anesthetic setup.

g. Extraction tray (Figure 1-27)

    i. Basic setup

    ii. Anesthetic setup

    iii. Retractors, elevators, and forceps

    iv. Sutures, suture scissors, and needle holders

    v. Disposable items

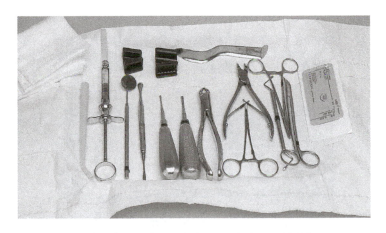

Figure 1-27 Tray setup for an uncomplicated extraction

h. Removable partial or full denture fabrication (Figure 1-28)

    i. Basic setup

    ii. Impression materials and trays

    iii. Lab items for denture fabrication

    iv. Disposable items

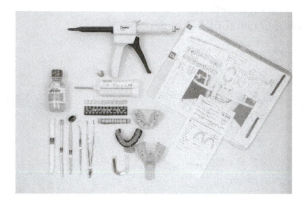

Figure 1-28 Tray setup for a final impression of a partial denture

i. Fluoride application tray

    i. Fluoride, trays, and timer

    ii. Disposable items

j. Incision and drainage tray

    i. Basic setup

    ii. Anesthetic setup

    iii. Bard Parker blade

    iv. Disposable items

k. dental dam (Figure 1-29)

    i. dental dam punch

    ii. forceps

    iii. frame

    iv. dental dam napkin

    v. beavertail burnisher

    vi. scissors

    vii. Wedjets ligature

    viii. clamp

    ix. dental dam material

    x. floss

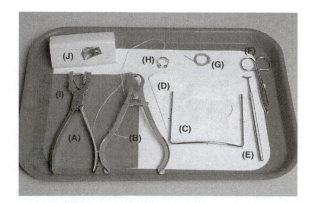

Figure 1-29 Dental dam tray setup (labeled). (A) Dental dam punch. (B) Forceps. (C) Frame. (D) Dental dam napkin. (E) Tucking instrument. (F) Scissors. (G) Wedjets ligature. (H) Clamp. (I) Dental dam material. (J) Floss.

    l. immediate dentures

m. impactions

        i. anesthetic syringe set up
        ii. periosteal elevators
        iii. curettes
        iv. appropriate forceps
        v. sutures/needles
        vi. surgical HVE tip
        vii. appropriate blades and blade holder
        viii. suture scissors
        ix. hemostats
        x. disposable items
        xi. basic set up
        xii. lip retractors

n. implants (Figure 1-30)

        i. intravenous sedation and local anesthetic setup
        ii. mouth mirror
        iii. surgical HVE tip
        iv. sterile gauze and cotton pellets
        v. irrigation syringe and sterile saline solution
        vi. low-speed handpiece
        vii. sterile template
        viii. sterile surgical drilling unit
        ix. scalpel and blades
        x. periosteal elevator
        xi. rongeurs
        xii. surgical curette
        xiii. tissue forceps and scissors
        xiv. cheek and tongue retractors
        xv. hemostat
        xvi. bite-block
        xvii. oral rinse
        xviii. Betadine
        xix. implant instrument kit
        xx. implant kit
        xxi. suture setup

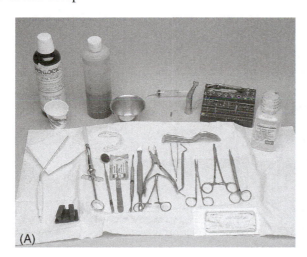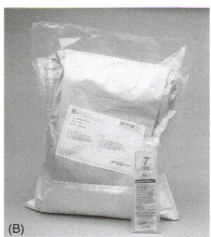

Figure 1-30 (A) Tray setup for implant surgery. (B) Surgical barrier kit.

o. initial/secondary impressions
   i. basic setup
   ii. HVE, air-water syringe tip
   iii. cotton rolls and gauze
   iv. custom tray
   v. impression material
   vi. lab knife
   vii. lab prescription
   viii. disinfectant and container

p. interceptive orthodontics

q. occlusal equilibration/adjustment (Figure 1-31)
   i. basic setup
   ii. cotton rolls and 2 × 2 gauze
   iii. saliva ejector, HVE tip, and air-water syringe
   iv. articulation forceps and articulating paper
   v. low-speed handpiece
   vi. diamond burs, discs, and stones
   vii. polishing wheels and discs

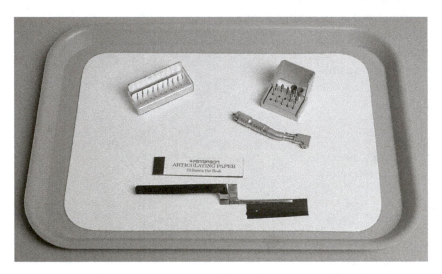

Figure 1-31 Tray set up for occlusal equilibration

r. oral examination
   i. basic setup
   ii. gauze 2 × 2s

s. oral prophylaxis (Figure 1-32)
   i. basic setup
   ii. saliva ejector, HVE tip, and air-water syringe
   iii. cotton rolls and gauze sponges
   iv. periodontal probe
   v. scalers: Jacquette and Shepherd's hook
   vi. curettes: Universal and Gracey
   vii. dental floss and dental tape
   viii. prophy angle – rubber cups and brushes
   ix. prophy paste

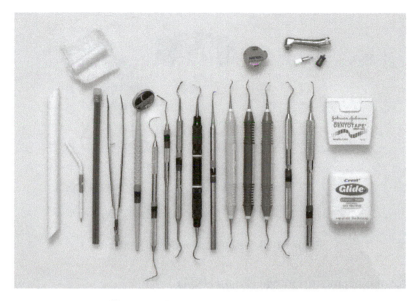

Figure 1-32 Tray setup for prophylaxis

t. periodontal procedures

    i. these will vary with each office.

u. periodontal surgical dressing placement/removal

    i. basic set up

    ii. periodontal surgical dressing

    iii. plastic instrument for festooning material around area to be dressed

v. root planning and curettage

    i. basic set up

    ii. scalers and curettes

    iii. disposable items

    iv. anesthetic syringe setup if needed

    v. Cavitron with various tips

w. rotary instruments

    i. slow speed with nosecone or contra angle

    ii. high speed with bur chuck if indicated

x. sealant application (Figure 1-33)

    i. basic setup

    ii. air-water syringe, HVE tips, and saliva ejector

    iii. rubber cup or brush

    vi. Dri-angles®

    v. low-speed handpiece with right-angle prophy attachment

    vi. prophy paste

    vii. dental dam setup

    viii. etchant and conditioner

    ix. sealant material

    x. applicators

    xi. bonding agent

    xii. during light

    xiii. articulating paper and forceps

    xiv. assorted burs and stones

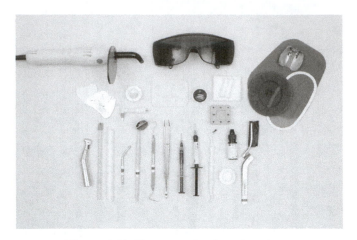

Figure 1-33 Tray setup for dental sealants

y. stainless steel crown placement/removal (Figure 1-34)

    i. basic setup
    ii. cotton rolls and gauze
    iii. HVE and saliva ejector
    iv. high-speed handpiece with selected burs
    v. low-speed handpiece with green stone and rubber abrasive wheel
    vi. spoon excavator
    vii. selection of stainless steel crowns
    viii. crown and collar scissors
    ix. contouring and crimping pliers
    x. mixing spatula, paper pad, and permanent cement
    xi. articulating paper and forceps
    xii. dental floss

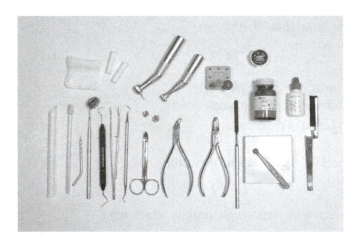

Figure 1-34 Tray setup for stainless steel crown placement

z. suture placement and removal

  a. temporary cementation

    i. provisional temporary to be placed
    ii. temporary cement (base and catalyst)
    iii. spatula and mixing pad
    iv. disposable items

    b. temporary restoration
        i. temporary cement (base and catalyst)
        ii. spatula and mixing pad
        iii. condenser and carver
        iv. matrix band and retainer with wedges
        v. basic set up
        vi. disposable items
    c. treatment of dry socket (Figure 1-35)
        i. local anesthetic setup
        ii. mouth mirror
        iii. irrigating syringe and warm sterile saline
        iv. surgical HVE tip
        v. surgical curettes
        vi. iodoform gauze or sponge material
        vii. cotton pliers
        viii. surgical scissors
    d. bleaching

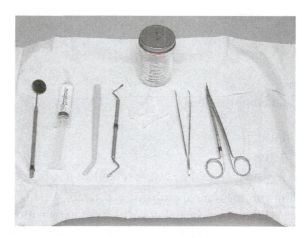

Figure 1-35 Tray setup for treatment of dry socket

C. When performing or assisting with intraoral procedures, the assistant should be familiar with the following:

1. Maintaining field of operation during dental procedures through the use of retraction, suction, irrigation, and drying.

2. Placing and removing cotton rolls using cotton forceps or other appropriate devices.

3. Assisting with and/or polishing teeth.

4. Assisting with and/or applying topical fluoride requires the assistant to choose the appropriate-size trays and proper fluoride. There are several types of fluorides, and each has its own use.

5. Assisting with and/or performing a vitality test requires that the assistant have the various vitality testing methods out and ready to record the results.

6. Assisting with and/or controlling minor bleeding after any surgical procedure requires the assistant to understand the clotting process and how to control bleeding through different methods such as pressure, tea bags, or other methods used in the office.

7. Assisting with, placing, and/or removing temporary cement requires the assistant to use an explorer or scaler to gently remove temporary cement supragingivally. Using floss to remove cement interproximally is also sometimes required.

8. Assisting with and/or applying and removing the dental dam.

9. Preparing, assisting with, and/or applying and removing matrix bands.

10. Assisting with and/or applying topical anesthetic to the site injection requires a general understanding of injection sites to include infiltration, mandibular block, and other injection sites.

11. Assisting with and/or monitoring the administration of nitrous oxide/oxygen analgesia requires the assistant to understand the concept of N_2O_2 sedation and its general effects on the patient. The patient is never left alone while under the influence of N_2O_2. General knowledge of the N_2O_2 equipment is a must in order to effectively assist the operator in the administration of the gas.

12. Identifying and exchanging rotary instruments in dental handpieces.

13. Use the concepts of four-handed dentistry and assisting with the following restorative procedures.
    a. administration of anesthetics
    b. cavity preparation and restoration
    c. crown and bridge restoration preparation, temporization, and cementation
    d. desensitization of the teeth
    e. endodontic therapy
    f. oral surgery
    g. fabrication of removable partial or full dentures
    h. fluoride application
    i. occlusal equilibration/adjustment
    j. occlusal registration
    k. oral examination and data collection
    l. oral prophylaxis
    m. periodontal procedures
    n. placement of sealants
    o. placement of stainless steel crowns
    p. postoperative treatment and complications
    q. implants
    r. suture placement and removal
    s. taking initial/secondary impressions

D. During patient management, the assistant should be aware of patient needs.

1. Demonstrate the ability to calm and reassure apprehensive patients. Often, a patient will become apprehensive, and usually it is because they fear the unknown. A brief explanation of the procedure and what to expect will go a long way in creating a calm atmosphere for the patient. Reassuring and checking on the patient throughout the procedure also helps alleviate apprehension.

2. Manage patients, including patients with special needs. At times, you will encounter a patient with special needs. A patient who may be developmentally disabled or physically disabled may need additional help when getting in and out of the dental chair. Having the patient's caregiver in the operatory can be a great help in both physically assisting the patient as well as mentally keeping the patient encouraged.

3. Monitor and record patient's response to drugs/medications. Patients have a natural anxiety when it comes to having dental treatment. These patients sometimes benefit from taking a premedication such as an antianxiety medication prior to their appointment. Also, **Nitrous Oxide Oxygen** sedation helps alleviate apprehension, and the patient must be monitored very closely. Nitrous Oxide Oxygen can bring the patient close to unconsciousness which is not the desired effect as patients can have their airway obstructed and suffocate if not monitored carefully. A patient should never fall asleep while under Nitrous Oxide Oxygen sedation. Also, a patient is never to be left alone during Nitrous Oxide Oxygen sedation. A patient who has taken antianxiety medication or who is under Nitrous Oxide Oxygen sedation must be monitored for airway obstruction and breathing difficulty. The patient may doze but must be able to take simple commands, and care must be taken to avoid injury to the patient. These patients must have help with getting in and out of the chair, and when the procedure is completed, aid must be given so the designated caregiver can take the patient home. A patient is never allowed to leave on their own after taking antianxiety medications. Nitrous Oxide Oxygen sedation is different in that the gas is cleared from the bloodstream after three minutes of pure oxygen. Only after adequate oxygen is given and the patient is fully recovered are they allowed to leave the treatment area. FYI: Nitrous tanks are always blue and oxygen tanks are always green. Keep tanks and equipment up to date and maintained.

Important Concepts to Know

1. Identify the armamentaria needed for all general and specialty practices such as oral surgery, endodontics, periodontics, prosthodontics, orthodontics, and pediatrics.
2. Demonstrate how to pass and receive instruments and armamentaria for all general dental procedures.
3. Demonstrate how to manage patients who have special needs and patients who may find dental procedures unusually stressful.
4. Understand patient responses regarding different medications and how to identify and record those responses.

Study Checklist

1. Review terminology as it relates to four-handed dentistry, chairside assisting, and patient management.
2. Read textbook chapters on four handed-dentistry and patient management
3. Review setup and treatment room preparation.
4. Review chairside restorative procedures.
5. Read textbook information on all general dental procedures and armamentarium.

Section II:
Chairside Dental Procedures –
Review Questions

Use the Answer Sheet found in Appendix A.

1. The _____ is the part of the instrument where the operator grasps or holds the instrument.
   a. shank
   b. handle
   c. nib
   d. working end

2. The basic setup consists of
   a. mouth mirror, periodontal probe, and explorer.
   b. mouth mirror, explorer, and spatula.
   c. cotton pliers, mouth mirror, and explorer.
   d. mouth mirror and explorer.

3. Explorers have which of the following characteristics?
   a. They are not used in diagnosis.
   b. They are useful in detecting subtle anomalies in tooth structures.
   c. They have a knife-like working end.
   d. They can be used to remove calculus on the inter-proximal surfaces of the teeth.

4. A spoon excavator
   a. is a hand instrument with a working end that is shaped like a spoon.
   b. is used to remove soft decay.
   c. is used when the operator does not want to create a pulpal exposure by using more aggressive decay removal techniques.
   d. all of the above

5. Amalgam condensers are used to
   a. carry amalgam to the preparation.
   b. pack amalgam into the preparation.
   c. mix mercury and alloy together to create amalgam.
   d. remove old amalgam material.

6. The operator is completing an amalgam restoration and needs to place detailed anatomy in the occlusal surface of the tooth. The instrument an assistant would pass to him would be which of the following?
   a. hoe
   b. hatchet
   c. carver
   d. condenser

7. An operator would like to smooth condensed amalgam on a filled tooth. Which instrument would the assistant pass to the operator?
   a. carver
   b. hatchet

c. hoe
d. burnisher

8. The best instrument to use to place and manipulate composite material would be
   a. condenser.
   b. carver.
   c. plastic instrument.
   d. chisel.

9. The assistant prepares a tray for a crown preparation. Which item would not likely be found on this tray?
   a. cord-retraction instrument
   b. basic setup
   c. ball burnisher
   d. diamond bur

10. The best way to remove loose interproximal cement on a newly cemented crown is by
    a. using a scaler.
    b. using an ultrasonic handpiece.
    c. using the air/water syringe.
    d. using a piece of floss with a knot tied in the middle.

11. A patient presents with pain on the lower right first molar. Which tray would be the most appropriate to place on the bracket table?
    a. endodontic
    b. pulp vitality testing
    c. crown prep
    d. extraction

12. The operator needs to remove set cement from a permanent crown. Which instrument would be the most appropriate to use?
    a. an ultrasonic handpiece
    b. a prophy cup and pumice
    c. a high-speed handpiece
    d. a lab bur

13. The high-speed contra-angle handpiece reaches speeds of _____.
    a. 225,000 rpm
    b. 400,000 rpm
    c. 495,000 rpm
    d. 665,000 rpm

14. Which of the following is NOT true about the slow-speed handpiece?
    a. is used to remove soft decay
    b. can be used to polish restorations and tooth material
    c. used for removal of decay on hard enamel
    d. comes with a variety of attachments

15. Which of the following does NOT apply to the laser handpiece?
    a. used for surgical procedures
    b. contains a light source through a fiber-optic cable
    c. can be used to cut, cauterize, or vaporize tissue
    d. requires water to operate

16. Why should the high-speed handpiece be sterilized after each patient use?
    a. It is the standard of care.
    b. The dentist is responsible for any patient illness.
    c. It extends the longevity of the handpiece.
    d. The high-speed handpiece is autoclavable.

17. Which of the following is NOT a type of carbide bur?
    a. round fissure
    b. tapered cross-cut fissure
    c. inverted cone fissure
    d. flame diamond

18. A mandrel is used to
    a. extend the bur length by 2 mm.
    b. attach polishing devices to the slow-speed handpiece.
    c. sharpen polishing stones.
    d. remove gross amounts of enamel.

19. When adjusting or polishing gold or amalgam restorations, the assistant should place which of the following items in the high-speed handpiece?
    a. stone or rubber point
    b. carbide bur
    c. diamond bur
    d. large round bur

20. Finishing strips are used to smooth which surfaces of the finished restoration?
    a. buccal and lingual
    b. mesial and distal
    c. facial and distal
    d. incisal and lingual

21. Rubber points and stones can be
    a. used one time and then discarded.
    b. used only outside the patient's mouth.
    c. sterilized and reused.
    d. sharpened when they become dull.

22. High-speed handpieces generally use which type of bur?
    a. latch type
    b. friction grip
    c. static
    d. concentrated

23. Amalgam placed in the cavity preparation is most often accomplished by using a
    a. burnisher.
    b. carver.
    c. condenser.
    d. amalgam carrier.

24. After placing amalgam into the cavity preparation, the operator will most likely use which instrument to compact the amalgam into the preparation?
    a. condenser
    b. burnisher
    c. carver
    d. compactor

25. Anatomy placed into the condensed amalgam can be accomplished by using which instrument?
    a. acorn burnisher
    b. articulator
    c. enamel hatchet
    d. hoe

26. If the operator asks for the assistant to provide an instrument to check the occlusion of a finished amalgam, which item would the assistant most likely hand the operator?
    a. carver
    b. articulating paper/holder
    c. burnisher
    d. wax bite

27. While assisting during an amalgam, which bur would most likely appear on the armamentarium tray?
    a. round carbide
    b. diamond bur
    c. fluted carbide
    d. white stone

28. Custom trays are designed to
    a. fit only the person they were made for to render a more accurate impression.
    b. provide comfort to the patient.
    c. be used with alginate only.
    d. be waterproof.

29. When desensitizing tooth structures, the tissue of the tooth that is treated is
    a. enamel.
    b. dentin tubules.
    c. pulpal.
    d. cementum.

30. An immediate denture is placed
    a. as soon as the patient arrives.
    b. immediately following extractions.
    c. right after it's fabricated in the office.
    d. only as a temporary until the permanent is fabricated.

31. A patient had an extraction preformed earlier in the day and returns complaining that the extraction site continues to bleed. The dentist would most likely ask the assistant to perform what action?
    a. Call 911.
    b. Attempt to control bleeding by applying pressure.
    c. Place an ice pack on the site and send the patient home.
    d. Send the patient to their medical doctor for a vitamin C injection.

32. In the "single-handed transfer," the assistant's hand is divided into two parts, which consist of
    a. thumb/finger and palm portions.
    b. fingertips and open hand.
    c. little finger area and thumb-finger area.
    d. fingertip and between finger portions.

33. The benefits of proper instrument transfer techniques include
    a. decreased needlestick injuries associated with the use of dental instruments.
    b. reduction in neck strain for the patient.
    c. patient comfort.
    d. decreased tactile sensitivity for the operator.

34. When transferring bulky instruments such as rubber dam forceps or surgical forceps, the best transfer method is the
    a. modified pen grasp.
    b. two-handed transfer.
    c. hidden syringe transfer.
    d. single-handed transfer.

35. When performing the single-handed transfer, the instrument being delivered is _____ to the instrument being retrieved.
    a. perpendicular
    b. opposite
    c. parallel
    d. at a right angle

36. The patient is receiving Nitrous Oxide Oxygen sedation during a procedure. You ask the patient if they are doing all right and get no response, but the patient seems to be breathing without any trouble. Is this a concern?
    a. Not usually. As long as the patient is breathing, it is all right for the patient to sleep.
    b. Yes. A patient should never be in a state in which they cannot respond to simple commands.
    c. It depends on what the operator deems appropriate.
    d. No. It's not a concern, as a patient who is unresponsive on Nitrous Oxide Oxygen is easier to work on than a patient who is responsive.

37. The dentist asks you to set up an operative tray for endodontic therapy on tooth #14. Which item would NOT appear on the tray?
    a. Gates-Glidden reamers
    b. spreader
    c. discoid-cleoid
    d. K-type files

38. The dentist asks you to set up an operative tray for a composite restoration on tooth #2 MOD. Which item would NOT appear on the tray?
    a. matrix band and wedges
    b. condenser
    c. a curing light
    d. Peeso reamers

39. While assisting, the assistant's chair should be _____ the operator's chair.
    a. higher than
    b. lower than
    c. even with
    d. at a right angle to

40. While preparing a tray for endodontic therapy, the dentist tells you that he will need to isolate the tooth for the procedure. In response to this request, what would you place on the tray?
    a. cotton rolls
    b. a dental dam, frame, and clamp
    c. gauze 2 × 2 squares
    d. a surgical suction tip

41. When preparing an anesthetic tray, the gauze 2 × 2 square is placed on the tray to
    a. dry the mucosa prior to placing topical anesthetic.
    b. wipe the end of the carpule prior to loading into the syringe.
    c. drying or isolating the tooth prior to giving the injection.
    d. wipe any anesthetic off the syringe needle prior to administering the injection.

42. A Tofflemire matrix band is NOT used for the following restoration:
    a. MO amalgam
    b. DO amalgam
    c. class V restoration
    d. MOD composite

43. The bur used most often during a crown preparation is
    a. 1157 carbide bur.
    b. cylindrical diamond bur.
    c. #6 round carbide friction grip bur.
    d. #8 round carbide slow-speed bur.

44. The dentist tells you to set up a matrix band and retainer to restore the upper right first bicuspid. The tooth you are restoring is which tooth?
    a. #2
    b. #3
    c. #4
    d. #5

45. When setting up a room for treatment on a patient who will be receiving Nitrous Oxide Oxygen sedation, the oxygen tank is which color?
    a. blue
    b. green
    c. black
    d. white

46. Asking the caregiver of a physically or mentally disabled patient to stay in the operatory can create the following situation:
    a. calm and reassure the patient
    b. create distress for the patient
    c. create a distraction for the operator
    d. lending a hand by keeping the patient entertained

47. For the right-handed operator, the transfer zone is located in which clock position?
    a. four and seven o'clock
    b. two and four o'clock
    c. seven and twelve o'clock
    d. twelve and two o'clock

48. The static zone is utilized for which type of dentistry?
    a. surgical procedures
    b. four-handed dentistry
    c. restorative procedures only
    d. six-handed dentistry

49. The intraoral examination consists of all of the following EXCEPT
    a. the dentist examining the inside of the patient's mouth.
    b. the dentist examining the patient's tongue.
    c. the assistant recording medications being taken by the patient.
    d. the dentist examining the patient's tonsils.

50. When setting up a procedure tray, how should the assistant set up the instruments on the tray?
    a. in reverse order
    b. in order of use
    c. in a random order; it doesn't really matter
    d. in order of largest to smallest

51. During dental treatment, what would be the most efficient way to retrieve an instrument out of the drawer or out of the treatment area?
    a. use a gloved hand
    b. use an overglove or remove the glove, use a bare hand, and don a new glove
    c. use the blue nitrile or heavy-duty housekeeping gloves
    d. use a gloved hand but wash the gloves prior to retrieving needed supplies

52. A circulating or second assistant is utilized during which kind of dentistry?
    a. four-handed
    b. six-handed
    c. recall
    d. stand-up

53. Where does the assistant sit in relation to the operator?
    a. four to six inches higher than the operator
    b. four to six inches lower
    c. four to six inches higher than the patient's chin
    d. even with the operator

54. Which of the following items would not be found on an amalgam tray?
    a. burnisher
    b. discoid-cleoid
    c. condenser
    d. plastic instrument

55. Which of the following items would not be found on a composite tray?
    a. Mylar strip
    b. acid etch
    c. cord-packing instrument
    d. curing light

56. Which item would not appear on a periodontal surgery tray?
    a. surgical blade
    b. periosteal elevator
    c. sutures
    d. lab knife

57. What color are the nitrogen tank and the oxygen tank in the dental office?
    a. blue, yellow
    b. blue, orange
    c. green, blue
    d. blue, green

58. Which zone matches up with region seven o'clock to twelve o'clock?
    a. transfer zone
    b. operator zone
    c. assisting zone
    d. static zone

59. Which of the following instruments would appear on an amalgam restoration tray?
    a. rongeurs
    b. burnisher
    c. curette
    d. prophy angle

Section II: Chairside Dental Procedures – Answers and Rationales

1. The _____ is the part of the instrument where the operator grasps or holds the instrument.

   b. handle

2. The basic setup consists of

   a. mouth mirror, periodontal probe, and explorer.

3. Explorers have which of the following characteristics?

   b. They are useful in detecting subtle anomalies in tooth structures.

4. A spoon excavator

   d. all of the above – A spoon excavator has two working ends with scoop-like working ends. It is used primarily to remove soft decay by hand so as not to create a pulpal exposure, which can occur by using a slow-speed round bur. It gives the operator more control and finesse when removing decay.

5. Amalgam condensers are used to

   a. carry amalgam to the preparation.

6. The operator is completing an amalgam restoration and needs to place detailed anatomy in the occlusal surface of the tooth. The instrument an assistant would pass to him would be which of the following?

   c. Carver – A condenser packs the amalgam into the prep, and hoes and hatchets are used to carve detail into the dentin or enamel in preparation for the amalgam or composite material.

7. An operator would like to smooth condensed amalgam on a filled tooth. Which instrument would the assistant pass to the operator?

   d. burnisher – A burnisher smoothes the restoration and seals the margins by burnishing the material against the margins of the preparation. A carver carves detail into the restoration, and hoes and hatchets assist in cutting the prep for the restoration.

8. The best instrument to use to place and manipulate composite material would be

   c. plastic instrument – Condensers are used to condense material into the prep, a carver is used to carve anatomy into restoration, and a chisel assists in cutting fine anatomy into the cavity preparation.

9. The assistant prepares a tray for a crown preparation. which item would not likely be found on this tray?

   c. Ball burnisher would not appear on a crown preparation tray. All other items such as a basic setup, cord retraction instrument, and a diamond bur would be found on a tray for a crown preparation.

10. The best way to remove loose interproximal cement on a newly cemented crown is by

    d. a piece of floss with a knot tied in the middle. This is very effective in removing a loose piece of interproximal cement after cementation of a crown. The other choices would be better for a piece of cement that has not been dislodged.

11. A patient presents with pain on the lower right first molar. Which tray would be the most appropriate to place on the bracket table?

    b. pulp vitality testing would be the logical tray to place on the bracket table. The other three trays – crown prep, extraction, and endodontic – would be premature when the doctor has not diagnosed the condition of the tooth.

12. The operator needs to remove set cement from a permanent crown. Which instrument would be the most appropriate to use?

    a. An ultrasonic handpiece is effective in completely removing excess cement from a seated permanent crown.

13. The high-speed contra-angle handpiece reaches speeds of _____.

    b. 400,000 rpm

14. Which of the following is NOT true about the slow-speed handpiece?

    c. used for removal of decay on hard enamel – The other choices are associated with a low-speed handpiece.

15. Which of the following does NOT apply to the laser handpiece?

    d. requires water to operate – Lasers do not require water to operate.

16. Why should the high-speed handpiece be sterilized after each patient use?

    a. It is the standard of care.

17. Which of the following is NOT a type of carbide bur?

    d. flame diamond

18. A mandrel is used to

    b. attach polishing devices to the slow-speed handpiece.

19. When adjusting or polishing gold or amalgam restorations, the assistant should place which of the following items in the high-speed handpiece?

    a. Stone (white) is used to polish amalgam and rubber points are used to polish gold.

20. Finishing strips are used to smooth which surfaces of the finished restoration?

    b. mesial and distal

21. Rubber points and stones can be

    c. sterilized and reused – You cannot sharpen them, and they are used inside the patient's mouth.

22. High-speed handpieces generally use which type of bur?

    b. friction grip

23. Amalgam placed in the cavity preparation is most often accomplished by using a

    d. amalgam carrier – Condensers pack the amalgam into the prep, carvers carve anatomy into the restoration, and burnishers smooth and seal the margins of the restoration.

24. After placing amalgam into the cavity preparation, the operator will most likely use which instrument to compact the amalgam into the preparation?

    a. condenser

25. Anatomy placed into the condensed amalgam can be accomplished by using which instrument?

    a. Acorn burnisher can be used as well as a carver for placing anatomy into a restoration.

26. If the operator asks for the assistant to provide an instrument to check the occlusion of a finished amalgam, which item would the assistant most likely hand the operator?

    b. articulating paper/holder

27. While assisting during an amalgam, which bur would most likely appear on the armamentarium tray?

    c. fluted carbide

28. Custom trays are designed to

    a. fit only the person they were made for to render a more accurate impression.

29. When desensitizing tooth structures, the tissue of the tooth that is treated is

    b. dentin tubules.

30. An immediate denture is placed

    b. immediately following extractions.

31. A patient had an extraction preformed earlier in the day and returns complaining that the extraction site continues to bleed. The dentist would most likely ask the assistant to perform what action?

    b. attempt to control bleeding by applying pressure

32. In the "single-handed transfer," the assistant's hand is divided into two parts, which consist of

    c. little finger area and thumb-finger area.

33. The benefits of proper instrument transfer techniques include

    a. decreased injuries associated with the use of dental instruments.

34. When transferring bulky instruments such as rubber dam forceps or surgical forceps, the best transfer method is the

    b. two-handed transfer.

35. When performing the single-handed transfer, the instrument being delivered is _____ to the instrument being retrieved.

    c. parallel

36. The patient is receiving Nitrous Oxide Oxygen sedation during a procedure. You ask the patient if they are doing all right and get no response, but the patient seems to be breathing without any trouble. Is this a concern?

    b. Yes. A patient should never be in a state in which they cannot respond to simple commands.

37. The dentist asks you to set up an operative tray for endodontic therapy on tooth #14. Which item would NOT appear on the tray?

    c. discoid-cleoid – This is used for amalgam restorations.

38. The dentist asks you to set up an operative tray for a composite restoration on tooth #2 MOD. Which item would NOT appear on the tray?

    c. A curing light is found on a composite tray.

39. While assisting, the assistant's chair should be _____ the operator's chair.

    a. higher than

40. While preparing a tray for endodontic therapy, the dentist tells you that he will need to isolate the tooth for the procedure. In response to this request, what would you place on the tray?

    b. a dental dam, frame, and clamp

41. When preparing an anesthetic tray, the gauze 2 × 2 square is placed on the tray to

    a. dry the mucosa prior to placing topical anesthetic.

42. A Tofflemire matrix band is NOT used for the following restoration:

    c. class V restoration

43. The bur used most often during a crown preparation is

    b. cylindrical diamond bur.

44. The dentist tells you to set up a matrix band and retainer to restore the upper right first bicuspid. The tooth you are restoring is which tooth?

    d. #5

45. When setting up a room for treatment on a patient who will be receiving Nitrous Oxide Oxygen sedation, the oxygen tank is which color?

    b. green

46. Asking the caregiver of a physically or mentally disabled patient to remain in the operatory can create the following situation:

    a. calm and reassure the patient

47. For the right-handed operator, the transfer zone is located in which clock position?

   a. four and seven o'clock transfer zone – Two and four is assisting zone, twelve and two is static zone, twelve and seven is operator zone.

48. The static zone is utilized for which type of dentistry?

   d. six-handed dentistry

49. The intraoral examination consists of all of the following EXCEPT

   c. the assistant recording medications being taken by the patient.

50. When setting up a procedure tray, how should the assistant set up the instruments on the tray?

   b. in order of use – Setting up instruments in order of use makes it easier for both the operator and the assistant to locate and utilize the instruments. It increases the efficiency of the procedure while helping both the assistant and the operator remain organized.

51. During dental treatment, what would be the most efficient way to retrieve an instrument out of the drawer or out of the treatment area?

   b. use an overglove or remove the glove, use a bare hand, and don a new glove – An overglove is the preferred way to retrieve instruments or supplies when sitting chairside. Removing the glove and then rewashing and regloving can be done, but is not practical.

52. A circulating or second assistant is utilized during which kind of dentistry?

   b. six-handed – A circulating or second assistant is an extra set of hands (hence, six-handed dentistry), and she/he is primarily used to retrieve supplies and instruments, retract, or mix materials when the first assistant is occupied chairside.

53. Where does the assistant sit in relation to the operator?

   a. four to six inches higher than the operator – This position give the assistant maximum visibility of the patient's oral cavity.

54. Which of the following items would not be found on an amalgam tray?

   d. plastic instrument – This instrument is usually found on the composite tray.

55. Which of the following items would not be found on a composite tray?

   c. cord-packing instrument – This instrument is used to pack retraction cord into the sulcus of the tooth and is found on a crown and bridge tray.

56. Which item would not appear on a periodontal surgery tray?

   d. lab knife – A lab knife doesn't leave the lab and is considered unsterile.

57. What color are the nitrogen tank and the oxygen tank in the dental office?

   d. blue, green

58. Which zone matches up with region seven o'clock to twelve o'clock.

   b. operating zone – This activity zone can be either for a right-handed operator.

59. Which of the following instruments would appear on an amalgam restoration tray?

   b. burnisher

Section III: Chairside Dental Materials (Preparation, Manipulation, Application)

This section of the General Chairside portion of the Certified Dental Assisting Examination consists of 9% or 11 questions of the 120 multiple-choice items. The questions related to this section of the General Chairside Dental Assisting Examination are based upon your knowledge of the following:

- Impression material
- Restorative materials
- Sedative/Palliative preparations
- Other dental materials

Key Terms

amalgam – an effective, long-lasting, and comparatively inexpensive material used for tooth restoration

cavity varnish – used to seal the dentin tubules to prevent acids, saliva, and debris from reaching the pulp

composite resin – material used to restore a tooth

dentin bonding – material that is used after the etch and conditioner. This material aids in the bonding of the composite restoration to the tooth.

etchant – substance used to roughen a surface before bonding

glass ionomer – permanent cementation material

periodontal dressing – bandage-like material applied to protect a surgical site as it heals

pit and fissure sealant – hard resin materials that are applied to the occlusal surface of carries-free posterior teeth to prevent decay

postextraction dressing – a paste or foam placed inside the extraction site socket to promote clotting and speed healing

reversible hydrocolloid – material used in the formation of dental impressions that can be converted from a gel to a solid and back to a gel based upon thermal reactions

sedative dressing – powder-and-liquid or two-paste system placed in the deepest part of the cavity preparation to provide an insulating base between the restoration and the tooth temporary or provisional restoration. A temporary or provisional restoration is placed in the interim between the preparation and placement of the final restoration. It is a temporary restoration and not meant as a long term solution.

Quick Review Outline

A. Impression Materials
   1. The dental assistant should be able to prepare, mix, and store the following materials for impressions.
      a. Irreversible hydrocolloid (alginate) – material used in the formation of dental impressions; setting of the material is accomplished by chemical reaction
      b. **Reversible hydrocolloid** (agar-gar) – material used in the formation of dental impressions that can be converted from a gel to a sol and back to a gel based upon thermal reactions.
      c. Elastomerics (polyether, polyvinylsiloxane) – a silicon-based material used to take final impressions
      d. Waxes
         i. pattern wax – used with a die to make a positive replica of a tooth
         ii. processing wax – types of waxes that are used to bead around trays, hold pieces of appliances together, or create a barrier to hold gypsum in place
         iii. impression wax – used to take bite registrations

> **NOTE** All impression materials are stored in a cool, dry area. Never store near heat or near water or moisture. Follow manufacturer's directions exactly when mixing impression materials.

B. Restorative

   1. The dental assistant should be able to prepare, mix, deliver, and store restorative materials

      a. **Amalgam** – most generally come in capsules that are compressed right before mixing. All scrap amalgam should be discarded in a sealed container with either fixer or mineral oil covering the scrap within it. Never discard in trash, Sharps container, or through the suction system. If mercury is spilled separately from the alloy powder, it is best to use a mercury spill kit. Never discard mercury in the trash, down the sink, in the Sharps container, or through the suction. Mercury is a heavy metal and can contaminate ground water supply if released into the environment. It is also toxic to humans.

      b. **Cements** – following manufacturer's recommendation, they are mixed on either a paper pad or a glass slab. Most cements are kept in a cool, dry area, while others are kept in the refrigerator to prolong shelf life.

      c. **Composite resin** – Most composites require a three-step system. Follow manufacturer's recommendation when using etch, primer, and bonding materials prior to composite placement. Most composites are cured with a light. Usually they are stored in a cool, dry place, but some may need to be refrigerated to prolong shelf life.

      d. **Dentin bonding** materials – usually included in the composite setup or can be used alone in certain applications.

      e. **Glass ionomers** – used as a permanent luting (cementing) agent. Some ionomers come in a powder/liquid mixing set, while others are contained in an automatic mixing syringe and are mixed at chairside just seconds before use. Most glass ionomers are stored in a cool, dry place, while others can be stored in the refrigerator to prolong shelf life.

      f. **Temporary restorative materials** – Similar to permanent cements, these come in a powder/liquid mixing set, while others are contained in an automatic mixing syringe and are mixed at chairside just seconds before use. Most temporary cements are stored in a cool, dry place, while others can be stored in the refrigerator to prolong shelf life.

      g. **Varnishes, bases, and liners** – Oftentimes, varnishes are in liquid form and are applied with a cotton pellet, while bases and liners are treated similarly to permanent and temporary cements. It is good to note that **cavity varnishes** are being used less in the dental field and have been replaced by other materials.

> **NOTE** **Each office and each operator will have their own preferred materials. It is up to the assistant to learn these preferences and use them with efficiency and confidence.**

   2. Prepare and/or seat aluminum temporary crowns

      a. select appropriate size

      b. using crown and bridge scissors and crimpers to trim and crimp to fit

      c. Temporary should fit both mesially and distally with no gaps and must fit snugly around the margin of the tooth. Sensitivity can occur if the margins of the preparation are exposed.

      d. cement with temporary cement

   3. The dental assistant should understand how to prepare and/or seat acrylic temporary crowns.

      a. Using alginate, take an impression prior to preparation.

      b. After the preparation has been cut, use acrylic or other designated material to create the temporary. A stent can be fabricated if the provisional is more than one unit. Trim excess acrylic and smooth. Cement the provisional with noneugenol cement. Eugenol does not interact with acrylic and begins to break down the acrylic, and therefore the temporary begins to lose its stability.

      c. Preformed acrylic temporary crowns are available for anterior teeth and can be filled with acrylic to simulate dentin. An alginate impression is not needed for this provisional.

C. Sedative/Palliative

   1. The dental assistant should be able to prepare, mix, and store sedative/palliative materials

      a. **Periodontal dressing** (surgical) – two-paste system used to protect surgical site during healing.

      b. **Postextraction dressing** – This can be a paste or foam placed inside the extraction-site socket to promote clotting and speed healing. This is usually used when dry socket occurs.

c. **Sedative dressing** – Powder-and-liquid or two-paste system placed in the deepest part of the cavity preparation to provide an insulating base between the restoration and the tooth. It can be permanent or temporary.

D. Other Dental Materials

1. The dental assistant should understand how to select and manipulate the various finishing, polishing, and cleaning agents. Polishing and finishing agents can come in many different applications. Sanding strips, sanding discs, paste that is applied to a rubber cup and then used with a slow-speed handpiece and applied to the tooth or restoration, special stones, and rubber points are all methods of application for polishing and finishing a restoration. Different operators will use different applications. It is the responsibility of the assistant to learn and make available these methods to the operator correctly and efficiently.

2. The dental assistant should understand how to prepare, mix, deliver, and store the following items.

   a. **bleaching or whitening agents** – stored in a cool, dry location and away from sunlight. Oftentimes, bleaching or whitening materials are stored in the refrigerator to prolong shelf life.
   b. **bonding agents** – multistep systems used in the restoration of a tooth using composite material. These materials can be either light or dual cure.
   c. **endodontic materials** – stored in a cool, dry location away from moisture and heat.
   d. **etchants** – used to remove the initial smear layer of a tooth in preparation of composite materials.
   e. **glass ionomer cements** – can be used in a powder/liquid or paste form. Generally used as a permanent cement and may contain fluoride.
   f. **pit and fissure sealants** – a two-step application consisting of an etchant and a sealer and used as a preventive measure to seal the occlusal surfaces of either primary or permanent nonrestored teeth. Usually stored in a cool, dry, moisture- and sunlight-free location.

Important Concepts to Know

1. Be familiar with how to mix, deliver, and store impression materials such as alginate, reversible hydrocolloid, elastomerics, and waxes.
2. Demonstrate how to prepare, mix, deliver, and store restorative materials such as amalgam, cements, composites, dentin bonding materials, glass ionomers, temporary restorative materials, varnishes, bases, and liners.
3. Review skills on preparing and seating temporary or provisional crowns.
4. Understand how to prepare, mix, and store sedative and palliative materials such as periodontal surgical dressing, postextraction dressings, and sedative dressings.
5. Demonstrate how to manipulate the various finishing, polishing, and cleaning agents such as finishing discs, white stones, rouge, and other materials used to polish or finish dental materials.
6. Demonstrate how to prepare, mix, deliver, and store dental materials such as bleaching agents, bonding agents, endodontic materials, etchants, glass ionomer materials, and pit and fissure sealant materials.

Study Checklist

1. Review terminology as it relates to restorative dental materials and their use.
2. Read textbook chapter on restorative dental materials.
3. Review skills for mixing and delivering various impression materials.
4. Review sections in periodontal chapter as it relates to periodontal dressings.
5. Review chapter sections as they relate to impression materials.

Section III:
Chairside Dental Materials – Review Questions

Use the Answer Sheet found in Appendix A.

1. Alginate is a/an _____ hydrocolloid
   a. reversible
   b. irreversible
   c. dual-cure
   d. light-sensitive

2. For operative dentistry, zinc phosphate cement is used
   a. to cement temporary crowns.
   b. as an alternative to a cavity liner.
   c. to cement permanent restorations.
   d. as a periodontal dressing.

3. Polycarboxylate cement is used
   a. as a base.
   b. as a liner.
   c. to cement permanent restorations.
   d. as a core buildup material.

4. Cavity varnish is
   a. applied before base material but after cavity liner.
   b. applied after cavity liner but before base material.
   c. never used with base material.
   d. always used with composite resin materials.

5. Zinc oxide eugenol is used as
   a. a base under composite restorations.
   b. an insulating base material.
   c. a permanent cements.
   d. a liner.

6. Glass ionomer contains _____, which is released slowly into the tooth structures.
   a. clove oil
   b. fluoride
   c. calcium
   d. phosphorus

7. _____ is used as a cavity liner or as pulp-capping material.
   a. Zinc phosphate
   b. Zinc oxide eugenol
   c. Calcium hydroxide
   d. Polycarboxylate cement

8. Zinc oxide eugenol contains _____, which soothes pulpal structures.
   a. fluoride
   b. clove oil
   c. calcium
   d. calcium hydroxide

9. When sizing an aluminum temporary crown, which of the following must occur?
   a. The crown must fit the area both mesially and distally.
   b. The crown must be trimmed and contoured to fit the preparation.
   c. The crown must not impinge on the gingiva.
   d. All of the above.

10. The preferred cement to use when cementing a temporary aluminum crown is
    a. zinc oxide eugenol cement.
    b. polycarboxylate cement.
    c. zinc phosphate cement.
    d. glass ionomer cement

11. Because of the exothermic properties of zinc phosphate, it is generally mixed
    a. on a paper pad.
    b. on a cool glass slab.
    c. in a dappen dish.
    d. with a metal spatula.

12. Amalgam is
    a. used primarily for posterior restorations or as a core buildup.
    b. economical to use.
    c. durable and will last several years.
    d. all of the above.

13. The operator asks you to prepare a material to line the base of a particularly deep cavity preparation. The best choice of material would be
    a. cavity varnish.
    b. calcium hydroxide.
    c. zinc phosphate.
    d. glass ionomer.

14. Cavity varnish is generally applied to the tooth so that which of the following occurs?
    a. insulation from pressure
    b. the tooth can be desiccated
    c. stimulation of secondary dentin
    d. seal dentin tubules and decrease sensitivity

15. The pulp-soothing component is zinc oxide eugenol is what material?
    a. calcium
    b. clove oil
    c. peroxide
    d. baking soda

16. To dissipate heat, zinc phosphate must be mixed with what?
    a. frozen mixing pad
    b. cooled mixing spatula
    c. waxed paper pad
    d. cooled glass slab

17. Glass ionomer contains _____, which is slowly released into the tooth.
    a. fluoride
    b. zinc oxide eugenol
    c. peroxide
    d. antibiotics

18. Luting agents are primarily used
    a. to seal dentin tubules.
    b. as a base.
    c. to stimulate secondary dentin.
    d. to cement permanent restorations.

19. Which of the following are characteristics of calcium hydroxide?
    a. used to stimulate reparative dentin
    b. is irritating to the pulp
    c. used to cement permanent restorations
    d. can be used for primary teeth only

20. Intermediate cements are expected to last at least _____ months.
    a. two
    b. three
    c. six
    d. nine

21. When/where is a periodontal surgical pack usually placed?
    a. over an extraction site
    b. around healing dental implants
    c. whenever teeth are temporarily splinted
    d. directly over a surgical site

22. On which of the following tissues would cavity varnish be placed?
    a. enamel
    b. dentin
    c. gingival
    d. none of the above tissues require varnish

Section III:
Chairside Dental Materials – Answers and Rationales

1. Alginate is an _____ hydrocolloid.

   b. **irreversible – Once alginate is mixed, it cannot revert to its original powder-and-liquid state.**

2. For operative dentistry, zinc phosphate cement is used

   c. **to cement permanent restorations – Zinc phosphate can be used to cement permanent crowns and is mixed on a cool glass slab. It is never used as a liner because of the irritation of phosphoric acid to the pulp and is not intended as a periodontal dressing.**

3. Polycarboxylate cement is used

   a. **as a base-because of its compatibility with amalgam and composite, it may be used as a nonirritating base under either of these materials.**

4. Cavity varnish is

   b. **applied after cavity liner but before base material-cavity varnish is applied in two thin coats to seal dentin tubules and reduce thermal sensitivity. It should be placed after a cavity liner to avoid sensitivity. It can be used with zinc phosphate or zinc oxide eugenol base materials but not with resin due to the incompatibility.**

5. Zinc oxide eugenol is used as

   b. **an insulating base material-zinc oxide eugenol can be used under amalgam restorations as an insulating base material. Because of the eugenol (clove oil) content, it is not compatible with composite materials. It is not strong enough to be used as a permanent cement or thin enough to be used as a liner.**

6. Glass ionomer contains _____, which is released slowly into the tooth structures.

   b. **fluoride-fluoride is contained in glass ionomer cements. It is slowly released into the tooth structures. Glass ionomers come in powder/ liquid, capsules, light cure, and paste depending on their intended use.**

7. _____ is used as a cavity liner or as pulp-capping material.

   c. **calcium hydroxide-calcium hydroxide is used as a cavity liner and as a pulp capping application. Calcium hydroxide provides the opportunity for reparative dentin to form within the tooth.**

8. Zinc oxide eugenol contains _____, which soothes pulpal structures.

   b. **clove oil-clove oil is the main component in eugenol. For centuries, clove oil has been used as a topical anesthetic and can provide comfort to dental tissues during the healing phase.**

9. When sizing an aluminum temporary crown, which of the following must occur?

   d. **all of the above-the crown must fit both mesially and distally to maintain spacing between the teeth while the permanent crown is being fabricated and cover the margins to prevent sensitivity.**

10. The preferred cement to use when cementing a temporary aluminum crown is

    a. **zinc oxide eugenol cement-this cement is the weakest cement of the four listed and can be removed easily while providing eugenol to soothe dental tissues.**

11. Because of the exothermic properties of zinc phosphate, it is generally mixed

    b. **on a cool glass slab-this procedure helps to keep the material cool while mixing which prolongs the working time which gives the assistant and operator more time to mix and seat.**

12. Amalgam is

    d. **all of the above-amalgam is strong and durable and for esthetic purposes used on posterior teeth, as a core buildup under crowns, and economical. There has been some controversy regarding the mercury in amalgam and health concerns but this theory has not been proven. Right now, it is just a theory.**

13. The operator asks you to prepare a material to line the base of a particularly deep cavity preparation. The best choice of material would be

    b. **calcium hydroxide is placed to stimulate secondary dentin.**

14. Cavity varnish is generally applied to the tooth so that which of the following occurs?

    d. **seal dentin tubules and decrease sensitivity – cavity varnish seals microscopic dentin tubules to prevents further sensitivity.**

15. The pulp-soothing component is zinc oxide eugenol is what material?

    b. **Clove oil or eugenol is added to the zinc oxide to soothe the pulpal structures.**

16. To dissipate heat, zinc phosphate must be mixed with?

    d. **Cooled glass slabs are used to mix zinc phosphate due to its high exothermic properties; this reduces the speed at which it sets.**

17. Glass ionomer contains _____, which is slowly released into the tooth.

    a. **fluoride**

18. Luting agents are primarily used

    d. to cement permanent restorations.

19. Which of the following are characteristics of calcium hydroxide?

    a. used to stimulate reparative dentin – Calcium hydroxide is placed in the deepest part of the cavity preparation and, over time, can aid in stimulating reparative dentin.

20. Intermediate cements are expected to last at least _____ months.

    c. six – Temporary cements are designed in strength and solubility to be effective for six months maximum. After that, they tend to wash out and become weak, compromising the preparation underneath.

21. When/where is a periodontal surgical pack usually placed?

    d. directly over a surgical site – A periodontal pack is placed directly over a surgical site to protect sutures that have been placed or to maintain tissue integrity while healing takes place.

22. On which of the following tissues would cavity varnish be placed?

    b. dentin – Varnish is placed on dentin to decrease its porosity and seal dentin tubules.

Section IV:
Lab Materials and Procedures

This section of the General Chairside portion of the Certified Dental Assisting Examination consists of 4% or 5 questions of the 120 multiple-choice items. The questions related to this section of the General Chairside Dental Assisting Examination are based upon your knowledge of the following:

- Selection and manipulation of laboratory materials
- Laboratory procedures

Key Terms

acrylic – a material that remains pliable and workable until a curing light is used to harden it
custom impression tray – a tray fabricated to meet a particular needs
dental waxes – used to take impression materials and aid in manufacture of appliances
gypsum – material used for pouring an impression to make a model

Quick Review Outline

A. Selection and Manipulation of Materials

    1. The dental assistant must know how to select and manipulate the various following **gypsum** products:

        a. plaster – also known as plaster of Paris. This is the weakest of the stones. It is generally used where detail and strength are not as important. Usually used to pour up study models, opposing models, mounting study models and casts, and for repairing casts. It is normally white in color.

        b. class I stone – This stone is three times as strong as plaster and used where strength is needed. It can be used for study models and working casts for partial and full dentures. It is normally yellow in color.

        c. class II stone – 30% stronger than class I stone and uses less water to incorporate its small, uniform parts. This stone is used for dies or where a strong model or cast is needed. This stone is usually light green in color.

        d. orthodontic stone – a mixture of plaster and class I stone that is stronger and can be used for orthodontic study models.

        e. quick-set stone – is used when an immediate model is needed and can be used during treatment because of its rapid setting time. This stone is usually pink in color.

    2. The dental assistant must know how to select and manipulate the following **dental waxes**.

        a. pattern wax – also known as inlay wax, which is used for constructing fixed and removable prostheses. Completely burns out at 900 degrees.

        b. processing wax – used for impressions (box wax or strips for the rim of trays), sticky wax (which is heated for bite registrations during denture fabrication), or orthodontic wax (placed over brackets that may be irritating to soft tissues).

    3. The dental assistant should be able to select and manipulate the various **acrylic** products or acrylic substitutes.

        a. Acrylic products usually have a powder base and a liquid catalyst. Mixing the liquid and powder in the given ratio lends strength and uniformity. Usually mixed in a paper or plastic cup with a metal spatula or tongue blade, it has a significant vapor, so good ventilation is always required.

    4. Properly store gypsum and acrylic products and dental waxes.

        a. Waxes should be stored at room temperature in a cool, dry location to avoid distortion.

        b. Gypsum and acrylic products are stored away from moisture in a cool, dry area away from the potential of getting wet.

B. Laboratory Procedures
1. Fabricating and evaluating diagnostic casts, including trimming and finishing
2. Debriding and polishing removable appliances and prostheses
3. Debriding and polishing fixed appliances and prostheses
4. Debriding and polishing complete/partial dentures.
   a. Cleaning complete or partial dentures varies with each office but usually starts with a bath in the ultrasonic (usually in a separate zip-top plastic bag) followed with a spray of disinfectant, and then the prostheses are rinsed completely again before being presented to the patient. If debris remains, a new toothbrush or denture brush may be used to gently scrub any remaining debris from the prostheses. This toothbrush or new denture brush may be rinsed thoroughly and passed on to the patient for future personal use.
5. Fabricating **custom impression trays**
   a. An alginate impression is taken of the arch in which the tray is going to be fabricated. After the model has been separated and trimmed, custom tray material is heated and manually formed around the model to conform to the patient's personal arch. A handle is constructed and attached, and then the edges are contoured and trimmed.
C. Laboratory equipment
   a. dental lathe or wheel
   b. a vacuform machine, which is used to make custom plastic trays for bleaching or fabricating orthodontic retainers or a stent
   c. model vibrator, which is used to eliminate bubbles and aid in pouring up dental models

Important Concepts to Know

1. Demonstrate how to properly to mix and prepare dental laboratory materials.
2. Demonstrate how to properly select and manipulate gypsum products.
3. Demonstrate how to properly select and manipulate dental waxes.
4. Demonstrate how to properly select and manipulate acrylic products or acrylic substitutes.
5. Demonstrate how to polish fixed and removable prostheses.
6. Demonstrate how to take, pour, and trim diagnostic casts.

Study Checklist

1. Review text chapter on dental lab materials.
2. Review text chapter on dental lab procedures.
3. Know terminology related to dental lab materials and procedures.

Section IV:
Lab Materials and Procedures – Review Questions

Use the Answer Sheet found in Appendix A.

1. _____ may be applied to the edge of the alginate trays to improve the fit of the tray.
   a. Boxing or utility wax
   b. Beading wax
   c. Orthodontic wax
   d. Pattern wax

2. A custom tray can be used only for the patient it was fabricated for.
   a. true
   b. false

3. Which of the following is true regarding a bite registration?
   a. can be made of wax or other putty-like material
   b. is used to articulate the maxilla and mandible
   c. is usually used by the lab to fabricate a permanent prostheses
   d. all of the above

4. Which of the following is true regarding elastomeric impressions?
   a. generally uses a base and catalyst
   b. is accurate and dimensionally stable
   c. can be used for crown and bridge fabrication
   d. all of the above

5. Gypsum materials include which of the following materials?
   a. plaster
   b. orthodontic stone
   c. quick-set stone
   d. all of the above

6. When sending a restorative case out for processing, it is not necessary to _____.
   a. place in a lab pan or other container to keep separate
   b. disinfect
   c. write up a detailed lab slip outlining instructions with the dentist's signature
   d. pour up the impression for the lab

7. Using a _____ will help ensure that no bubbles are created while pouring an impression.
   a. lab engine
   b. vibrator
   c. lab knife
   d. rolling motion with your hand

8. When trimming study models, the heels of the model are trimmed at _____ degrees.
   a. 30
   b. 45
   c. 95
   d. 115

9. Orthodontic stone is a mixture of _____ and _____.
   a. class II stone and quick-set stone
   b. class I stone and plaster
   c. plaster and calcium carbonate
   d. quick-set stone and plaster

10. Inlay wax is burned out of the dye at temperatures above _____ degrees F.
    a. 300
    b. 450
    c. 600
    d. 900

11. When a plaster model is curing, it will undergo a(n) _____ effect.
    a. endothermic
    b. exothermic
    c. reactionary
    d. binary

12. When fabricating a custom stent or bleach tray, the best way to accomplish this is by using a _____
    a. lab wheel.
    b. vacuform.
    c. lab engine.
    d. Cerec machine.

13. To polish acrylic dentures prior to delivery, a _____ can be used.
    a. lab engine
    b. lab wheel
    c. lab knife
    d. lab lathe

14. When pouring up an impression for a die, the best stone to use is _____
    a. class I stone.
    b. class II stone.
    c. quick-set stone.
    d. orthodontic stone.

15. Which type of wax is used in fabrication of a denture?
    a. utility wax
    b. baseplate wax
    c. casting wax
    d. bite registration wax

16. Type III stone that is used for lab procedures is most commonly is called which mix?
    a. orthodontic model stone
    b. laboratory stone
    c. high-strength die stone
    d. impression plaster

Section IV:
Lab Materials and Procedures –
Answers and Rationales

1. _____ may be applied to the edge of the alginate trays to improve the fit of the tray.

   a. **boxing or utility wax – Utility wax ropes are used around the periphery of the alginate tray to extend the length of the alginate tray or to provide a better fit around the vestibular areas.**

2. A custom tray can be used only for the patient it was fabricated for.

   a. **true – Because a custom tray is fabricated using the patient's study models, it is a custom fit for that particular patient and can be used for that patient only.**

3. Which of the following is true regarding a bite registration?

   d. **all of the above – Bite-registration material is used to articulate the bite between the maxillary and mandibular arches. Wax, polyvinylsiloxane impression material, or other putty-like materials may be used.**

4. Which of the following is true regarding elastomeric impressions?

   d. **all of the above – Polyvinylsiloxane impression material is used to take impressions for fixed and removable prostheses. It is provided in a base and catalyst and mixed just before placement in the mouth. PVS impression material is very dimensionally stable and does not require an immediate pour in stone or plaster.**

5. Gypsum materials include which of the following materials?

   d. **all of the above – Gypsum materials are used to create a positive reproduction created by the impression material. Gypsum products include plasters and stones.**

6. When sending a restorative case out for processing, it is not necessary to _____.

   d. **pour up the impression for the lab – Unless its an alginate impression, it is not necessary for the assistant to pour up an impression prior to it being sent out for processing. The lab usually prefers to pour its own cases.**

7. Using a _____ will help ensure that no bubbles are created while pouring an impression.

   b. **vibrator – This is used to gently vibrate the bubbles out of the impression material while it is being poured up.**

8. When trimming study models, the heels of the model are trimmed at _____ degrees.

   d. **115 degrees is the angle at which the heel or the back corners of the study model are trimmed.**

9. Orthodontic stone is a mixture of _____ and _____.

   b. **class I stone and plaster – This creates a harder, more durable stone for orthodontic casts.**

10. Inlay wax is burned out of the die at temperatures above _____ degrees F.

    d. **900 – Inlay or pattern wax is placed inside the die to create a positive impression of whatever dental item you are trying to reproduce. It is then burned out and the mold is left. This is where the porcelain or metals are poured to create the dental prostheses. This also known as the lost-wax technique.**

11. When a plaster model is curing, it will undergo a(n) _____ effect.

    b. **exothermic – Heat is given off during the curing process. When the model is cool to the touch, it is safe to break apart from the impression.**

12. When fabricating a custom stent or bleach tray, the best way to accomplish this is by using a _____.

    b. **vacuform – This machine heats the plastic and then forms it to the model by way of suction.**

13. To polish acrylic dentures prior to delivery, a _____ can be used.

    b. **A dental lathe or lab (rag) wheel can be used in conjunction with fine pumice to smooth rough areas on acrylic or porcelain. It is never used on gold. A special rouge and soft buffing wheel are used for gold.**

14. When pouring up an impression for a die, the best stone to use is _____.

    b. **class II stone – This stone has very small uniform parts, which make it a strong stone for this type of application.**

15. Which type of wax is used in fabrication of a denture?

    b. **baseplate wax – This wax is used in the fabrication of dentures.**

16. Type III stone that is used for lab procedures is most commonly is called which mix?

    b. **laboratory stone – This stone is usually yellow in color and is used for most lab procedures.**

Section V:
Patient Education and Oral Health Management

This section of the General Chairside portion of the Certified Dental Assisting Examination consists of 10% or 12 questions of the 120 multiple-choice items. The questions related to this section of the General Chairside Dental Assisting Examination are based upon your knowledge of the following:

- Oral health information
- Pre- and posttreatment instructions
- Plaque-control techniques
- Nutrition

Key Terms

autoimmune – immune response to one's own body tissue

bacteriostatic – inhibition of bacterial growth

bruxism – grinding of the teeth

carbohydrates – nutrient found in fruits, grains, legumes, and some vegetable roots

caries – tooth decay; cavities

crossbite – abnormal relationship of a tooth or a group of teeth in one arch to the opposing teeth in the other arch

distocclusion – the mandibular teeth occlude distally to their normal relationship to the maxillary teeth

disclosing agent – material that, when applied to teeth, will show the plaque buildup

exfoliate – to shed

fluoride – mineral essential to healthy bones and teeth

mesiocclusion – the mandibular teeth occlude mesially to their normal relationship to the maxillary teeth

open bite – abnormal vertical space between mandibular and maxillary teeth plaque acid attack this attack can last up to 20 minutes and occurs when carbohydrate sugars are introduced into the mouth. The bacteria in the mouth uses the carbohydrate sugars as food and the byproduct given off by the bacteria is in the form of plaque acid. This acid demineralized and damages the enamel of the teeth and manifests itself in the form of decay.

succedaneous teeth – permanent teeth

xerostomia – dry mouth

Quick Review Outline

A. Knowledge of general oral health information

  1. Implement patient education in the following areas:

    a. The dental assistant should understand the functions of the primary and permanent teeth and the relationship of the supporting structures.

      i. The permanent dentition has 32 teeth (12 molars, 8 premolars, 4 cuspids, 4 lateral incisors, 4 central incisors).

      ii. The primary dentition has 20 teeth (8 molars, 4 cuspids, 4 lateral incisors, 4 central incisors).

      iii. The periodontium consists of those tissues that support tooth function such as the gingiva, alveolar bone, periodontal ligament, and cementum.

    b. understanding the etiology or origin of dental disease such as decay and periodontal disease

      i. Plaque acid forms from the bacteria in plaque. The plaque consumes the sugars in carbohydrates and releases plaque acid, which destroys the surrounding hard tissues of the tooth and causes tooth decay.

      ii. Poor oral hygiene contributes to the formation of plaque acids, which leads to gum disease as well as tooth decay.

      iii. Neglecting regular maintenance of teeth and the surrounding tissues also plays a role in dental disease.

      iv. Personal oral habits such as smoking, chewing tobacco, and a high-carbohydrate diet also cause higher incidences of decay and periodontal disease.

c. the stages of eruption and exfoliation of the teeth (Tables 1-1 and 1-2)
  i. Teeth begin developing at approximately six weeks in utero.
  ii. Formation of tooth buds leads to development of primary and succedaneous teeth. (Note: **Succedaneous teeth** are those teeth that follow the exfoliation of other teeth. Bicuspids and third molars are not succedaneous teeth, as they arrive in the mouth independently and do not follow teeth of the same type.)
  iii. Tooth buds mature and develop distinct shapes during the apposition and calcification stage.
  iv. Primary teeth begin to **exfoliate** at approximately six years of age when succedaneous teeth begin to erupt.

Table 1-1 Eruption and Exfoliation Dates for Primary Teeth

Tooth	Eruption Date (Months)	Exfoliation Date (Years)	Maxillary Order
Central incisor	6–10	6–7	#1
Lateral incisor	9–12	7–8	#2
Canine	16–22	10–12	#4
First molar	12–18	9–11	#3
Second molar	24–32	10–12	#5
Central incisor	6–10	6–7	#1
Tooth	**Eruption Date (Months)**	**Exfoliation Date (Years)**	**Mandibular Order**
Lateral incisor	7–10	7–8	#2
Canine	16–22	9–12	#4
First molar	12–18	9–11	#3
Second molar	20–32	10–12	#5

Table 1-2 Eruption Dates for the Maxillary and Mandibular Permanent Teeth

Tooth	Eruption Date (Years)	Order of Eruption (Maxillary)
Central incisor	7–8	#2
Lateral incisor	8–9	#3
Canine	11–12	#6
First premolar	10–11	#4
Second premolar	11–12	#5
First molar	6–7	#1
Second molar	12–13	#7
Third molar	17–21	#8
Tooth	**Eruption Date (Years)**	**Order of Eruption (Mandibular)**
Central incisor	6–7	#2
Lateral incisor	7–8	#3
Cuspid	9–10	#4
First premolar	10–11	#5
Second premolar	11–12	#6
First molar	6–7	#1
Second molar	11–13	#7
Third molar	17–21	#8

d. Angle's classifications and other malocclusion
  i. class I – **neutroclusion** the lower teeth of the mandible rest behind the top teeth of the maxilla. This is the condition in which the anteroposterior occlusal relations of the teeth are normal.
  ii. class II – **distoclusion** – This occurs when the mandibular teeth occlude distally to their normal relationship to the maxillary teeth. Overjet or overbite is common.
  iii. class III – **mesiocclusion** – This occurs when the mandibular teeth occlude mesially to their normal relationship to the maxillary teeth. Edge-to-edge bite or underbite is common.
  iv. **overbite** – Vertical distance between upper and lower anterior teeth.
  v. **crossbite** – Maxillary teeth are positioned lingual to the mandibular teeth; this may occur unilaterally or bilaterally.
  vi. **openbite** – Abnormal vertical space between mandibular and maxillary teeth; most frequent in anterior area.
e. understanding the functions of saliva
  i. moisten food
  ii. wash away plaque and food debris
  iii. aid in speech
f. the advantages and disadvantages of restorative materials
g. the effects of systemic disease on the healing process
  i. **Autoimmune** diseases can impede the healing process due to the fact that the body is continually being attacked by its own immune system. Dental surgery and gum disease can take an even greater toll on a body that is already struggling to keep up with daily tissue turnover.
  ii. Cancer treatment can create barriers to healing due to energy required for recovering during the cancer-treatment process. During cancer treatment, patients suffer from **xerostomia** (dry mouth) and undernutrition, which can further complicate oral hygiene efforts.
  iii. A variety of medications for different medical conditions such as epilepsy, diabetes, hypertension, and heart conditions can create gingival hyperplasia and make it difficult to maintain adequate oral health.
  iv. Poor nutrition can play a significant role in the process of healing. The body requires sufficient amounts of vitamin C and calcium, just to name a few, during the healing of oral tissues. When adequate nutrition is not obtained, healing can slow dramatically or not occur at all.
h. It is important to understand the special dental health needs of various populations due to physical status, age, or disabilities.
  i. geriatric population
  ii. pediatric population
  iii. chronically ill
  iv. terminally ill
  v. temporary illnesses
  vi. special needs
  vii. physically disabled
i. The dental assistant should understand personal oral habits that may compromise oral health.
  i. **bruxism** (grinding of teeth)
  ii. thumb or finger sucking
  iii. tongue thrusting
  iv. tobacco chewing
  v. nail biting
  vi. smoking

2. It is important for the assistant to be able to explain procedures and services being delivered and their consequences to the patient and/or family.

   a. Patients and their families should be able to understand the outcomes of various procedures performed by the office. An extraction, a crown preparation, or any other procedure usually carries with it postoperative outcomes either with the procedure itself or medications that are taken following the treatment. It is beneficial for the assistant to be able to relay that information to the patient or a family member if it is needed.

3. The dental assistant should be able to explain the effects of the various types of **fluoride**, advantages and disadvantages of various types of fluoride administration, and the dangers and outcomes of overdosage.

   a. advantages

      i. remineralization of tooth structure
      ii. **bacteriostatic**
      iii. decreases cold sensitivity
      iv. prevention of **caries** formation

   b. disadvantages

      i. can be fatal if overdosed
      ii. some formulas of fluoride (Acidulated Phosphate Fluoride) may microetch porcelain veneers
      iii. some varieties may have an offensive taste
      iv. can cause stomach upset and nausea if swallowed

   c. recommended dosage

      i. in drinking water: 1 part per million (ppm)
      ii. for topical, follow manufacturer's recommendation
      iii. for supplements, follow the pharmacy/manufacturer/practitioner recommendations

B. The assistant should know how to deliver pre- and posttreatment instructions.

1. The dental assistant should be able to provide and explain to the patient pre- and posttreatment instructions, including instruction on prescribed medications as well as what to expect after treatment.

   a. Both written and verbal instructions can aid the patient in homecare.
   b. Written instructions give the patient a form of reference to look back on during the healing phase.

2. The assistant should be able to instruct the patient in how to care for removable and nonremovable appliances. They should be well versed in helping the patient increase oral hygiene health, speed healing time, and preserve the life of their prostheses.

C. The dental assistant should understand plaque-control techniques

1. How to evaluate the patient's oral health care status and habits

2. How and when to provide preventive oral health care information to the patient based on individual needs

3. Instructing the patient in appropriate toothbrush selection and brushing techniques

4. The assistant should be able to select and use plaque **disclosing agents** to assist in patient education.

5. The assistant should be able to assist the patient in selecting and using oral hygiene devices such as brushes, floss, interdental aids, oral rinses, and irrigating devices.

6. The assistant should be confident in evaluating the patient's progress in and response to homecare therapy on an ongoing basis.

D. The dental assistant should understand basic nutrition.

1. The assistant should be able to provide instruction and evaluate basic nutritional needs of individual patients as they relate to dental health.

2. The assistant should be able to explain to the patient the relationship of **carbohydrates** to the development of dental caries, also known as the plaque acid attack.

Important Concepts to Know

1. Understand oral health information such as the functions of primary and permanent teeth and their stages of eruption and exfoliation.
2. Explain the etiology or origin of dental disease.
3. Understand the classifications and importance of occlusion.
4. Explain the functions of saliva.
5. Explain the advantages and disadvantages of various restorative materials.
6. State the effects of systemic disease of the healing process.
7. Understand the various special needs of diverse populations.
8. Be able to deliver pre- and postoperative care instructions and explain outcomes to both patients and their families.
9. Understand plaque-control techniques and evaluation of patient oral hygiene status.
10. Comprehend basic nutrition as it relates to the needs of individual patients.

Study Checklist

1. Review text chapter on nutrition.
2. Review text chapter on embryology.
3. Review text information on plaque control, fluoride, and oral hygiene.
4. Understand basic terminology as it relates to nutrition, embryology, and plaque control.
5. Review text regarding special needs patients.

Section V:
Patient Education and Oral Health Management –
Review Questions

Use the Answer Sheet found in Appendix A.

1. Which oral hygiene device should the dental assistant recommend to the patient who has a fixed bridge?
   a. denture brush
   b. floss threader
   c. mouth rinse
   d. toothpick

2. Abrasion of the teeth may occur from using a _____
   a. hard-bristled toothbrush.
   b. heavy waxed dental floss.
   c. medium-bristle toothbrush.
   d. water-irrigating device.

3. The type of bone that supports the teeth is called _____
   a. cortical bone.
   b. periodontal bone.
   c. alveolar bone.
   d. attached bone.

4. Angle's classification is based on the
   a. shape of the maxilla.
   b. relationship between the first molars and the orbit of the eye.
   c. relationship between the maxillary and mandibular first molars.
   d. number of teeth in the mandible.

5. How many bicuspids are in the primary dentition?
   a. two
   b. four
   c. six
   d. none

6. Which part of the tooth forms first?
   a. crown
   b. root
   c. pulp
   d. dentin

7. The following fluoride can etch porcelain veneers:
   a. acidulated phosphate
   b. stannous fluoride
   c. sodium fluoride
   d. systemic fluoride

8. Bruxism can cause the posterior teeth to appear_____
   a. yellow.
   b. flattened.
   c. to have sharp points on the facial surface.
   d. mottled.

9. After receiving an epinephrine-containing anesthetic, the patient complains that his heart rate has increased and he feels anxious. The best course of action is to _____
   a. call 911.
   b. administer oxygen.
   c. tell the patient this is normal and it will pass.
   d. place the patient in the subsupine position and monitor breathing.

10. After reviewing the medical history of your patient, you notice she is taking hydrochlorothiazide (HCTZ). This is an indication that the patient is controlling _____
    a. epilepsy.
    b. high blood pressure.
    c. angina.
    d. migraines.

11. If your patient indicates that he is allergic to penicillin, it is best to substitute _____ for antibiotic treatment.
    a. Amoxicillin
    b. Clindamycin
    c. Keflex
    d. Pen VK

12. It is best not to give _____ to a patient who has a history of stomach ulcers or other disorders.
    a. OxyContin
    b. ibuprofen
    c. Tylenol with codeine
    d. hydrocodone

13. The best item to use to indicate areas of missed brushing on children is _____
    a. floss.
    b. disclosing tablets.
    c. fluoride drops.
    d. toothpaste.

14. The teeth in the permanent and primary dentition responsible for grinding and chewing food are referred to as _____
    a. incisors.
    b. bicuspids.
    c. cuspids.
    d. molars.

15. Primary central incisors begin to appear at _____
    a. 1–2 months of age.
    b. 5–6 months of age.
    c. 1 year of age.
    d. 18 months of age.

16. _____ are found mainly in fruits, grains, and vegetables and _____ are found in processed foods such as jelly, bread, crackers, and cookies.
    a. Proteins, carbohydrates
    b. Complex carbohydrates, fats
    c. Complex carbohydrates, simple sugars
    d. Proteins, simple sugars

17. Inflammation of the supporting tissues of the teeth that begins with _____ can progress into the connective tissue and alveolar bone that supports the teeth and becomes _____
    a. gingivitis, glossitis.
    b. periodontitis, gingivitis.
    c. gingivitis, periodontitis.
    d. gingivitis, gangrene.

18. The eating disorder that can easily be recognized in the dental office by severe wear on the lingual surface of the teeth caused by stomach acid from repeated vomiting is
    a. bulimia.
    b. binge eating.
    c. anorexia nervosa.
    d. female triathlon athlete.

19. The patient's record indicates that the status of the gingival tissue is bulbous, flattened, punched out, and cratered. This statement describes
    a. gingival color.
    b. gingival contour.
    c. consistency of the gingiva.
    d. surface texture of the gingiva.

20. Gum disease that involves red and edematous tissues and slight bone loss is referred to as
    a. gingivitis, glossitis.
    b. gingivitis, slight periodontitis.
    c. gingivitis, moderate periodontitis.
    d. gingivitis, severe periodontitis.

21. Malocclusion is best described as which situation?
    a. the abnormal relationship between the maxilla and mandible
    b. a high susceptibility to caries
    c. a class I occlusion
    d. difficulty with speech

22. Class I occlusion is also referred to as which condition?
    a. distoclusion
    b. mesiocclusion
    c. neutroclusion
    d. retrognathic

23. Patients undergoing cancer treatment such as chemotherapy and radiation can suffer which of the following symptoms?
    a. xerostomia
    b. no appetite
    c. increased caries activity
    d. The cancer patient can have any of these symptoms during treatment.

24. Which substance do plaque bacteria feed on to produce plaque acid?
    a. fats
    b. carbohydrate sugars
    c. proteins
    d. amino acids

25. Smoking can contribute to which of the following dental problems?
    a. oral cancer
    b. slow healing after dental surgery
    c. periodontal disease
    d. any of the above

26. Involuntary grinding of the teeth is referred to as what?
    a. attrition
    b. abrasion
    c. bruxism
    d. bulimia

27. Carbohydrates are primarily derived from which food group?
    a. proteins
    b. dairy
    c. fats and oils
    d. breads and cereals

28. Foods that break down in the mouth into simple sugars and can be used by the bacteria to cause dental caries are referred to as which of the following?
    a. cariogenic
    b. nutrient dense
    c. cariostatic
    d. insoluble

29. Systemic fluoride can be found in
    a. topical fluoride.
    b. fluoride rinses.
    c. fluoridated water.
    d. disclosing tablets.

Section V:
Patient Education and Oral Health Management –
Answers and Rationales

1. What oral hygiene device should the dental assistant recommend to the patient who has a fixed bridge?

   b. floss threader – This is a thin plastic loop that can be threaded under the pontic to remove debris from under the bridge and around the abutment tissues.

2. Abrasion of the teeth may occur from using a _____.

   a. hard-bristled toothbrush – Daily use of a hard-bristled toothbrush will cause abrasion and recession after prolonged use.

3. The type of bone that supports the teeth is called

   c. alveolar bone – This is the spongy bone that sits between the two cortical plates where the roots of the teeth are embedded.

4. Angle's classification is based on the

   c. relationship between the maxillary and mandibular first molars.

5. How many bicuspids are in the primary dentition?

   d. none – There are no bicuspids in the primary dentition.

6. Which part of the tooth forms first?

   a. crown

7. The following fluoride can etch porcelain veneers:

   a. acidulated phosphate – This fluoride can microetch porcelain products such as veneers or crowns with continued use.

8. Bruxism can cause the posterior teeth to appear_____.

   b. flattened – The repeated grinding of the teeth can cause the posterior as well as anterior teeth to become flattened.

9. After receiving an epinephrine containing anesthetic, the patient complains that his heart rate has increased and he feels anxious. The best course of actions is to _____.

   c. tell the patient this is normal and it will pass – Also known as an "epinephrine rush," this occurs when the vessels are nicked and anesthetic is injected directly into the bloodstream. It passes very quickly, and the patient should be told this to prevent anxiousness.

10. After reviewing the medical history of your patient, you notice she is taking hydrochlorothiazide (HCTZ). This is an indication that the patient is controlling _____.

    b. high blood pressure – HCTZ is the generic drug used to treat patients who have high blood pressure. This medication is a diuretic that helps prevent the body from absorbing too much salt, which can cause fluid retention that oftentimes results in high blood pressure or hypertension.

11. If your patient indicates that he is allergic to penicillin, it is best to substitute _____ for antibiotic treatment.

    b. Clindamycin – This is a safe antibiotic to use for patients who are allergic or sensitive to the "cillin" groups. All the other medications listed contain some form of penicillin.

12. It is best not to give _____ to a patient who has a history of stomach ulcers or other disorders.

    b. ibuprofen – Also known as Advil or Motrin by brand name; causes stomach and intestinal upset.

13. The best item to use to indicate areas of missed brushing on children is _____.

    b. disclosing tablets – These are orange or red tablets or liquid drops that are administered to children to detect where they have missed brushing. This tablet is chewed and swished and then expectorated into the sink. The disclosing solution adheres to plaque and then can be brushed off.

14. The teeth in the permanent and primary dentition responsible for grinding and chewing food are referred to as _____.

    d. molars – These are posterior teeth with broad, flat, chewing surfaces designed to grind food prior to swallowing.

15. Primary central incisors begin to appear at _____.

    b. 5–6 months of age – These are most likely the first teeth you see in a child's dentition.

16. _____ are found mainly in fruits, grains, and vegetables and _____ are found in processed foods such as jelly, bread, crackers, and cookies.

    c. Complex carbohydrates, simple sugars

17. Inflammation of the supporting tissues of the teeth that begins with _____ can progress into the connective tissue and alveolar bone that supports the teeth and becomes _____.

    c. gingivitis, periodontitis

18. The eating disorder that can easily be recognized in the dental office by severe wear on the lingual surface of the teeth caused by stomach acid from repeated vomiting is:

    a. bulimia – This an eating disorder in which the individual eats and then vomits.

19. The patient's record indicates that the status of the gingival tissue is bulbous, flattened, punched out, and cratered. This statement describes:

    b. gingival contour – Contour describes the shape and appearance of the tissue.

20. Gum disease that involves red and edematous tissues and slight bone loss is referred to as

    b. gingivitis, slight periodontitis.

21. Malocclusion is best described as which situation?

    a. the abnormal relationship between the maxilla and mandible

22. Class I occlusion is also referred to as which condition?

    c. neutroclusion – The teeth are resting in a neutral position with the maxillary teeth over the mandibular teeth, with the anterior mandibular teeth nestled behind the maxillary teeth with no evidence of overjet or overbite.

23. Patients undergoing cancer treatment such as chemotherapy and radiation can suffer which of the following symptoms?

    d. The cancer patient can have any of these symptoms during treatment.

24. Which substance does plaque bacteria feed on to produce plaque acid?

    b. carbohydrate sugars

25. Smoking can contribute to which of the following dental problems?

    d. any of the above

26. Involuntary grinding of the teeth is referred to as what?

    c. bruxism – Grinding causes wearing away of the incisal and occlusal surfaces of the teeth. A night guard is usually recommended for this.

27. Carbohydrates are primarily derived from which food group?

    d. breads and cereals – Carbohydrates also come fruits and vegetables.

28. Foods that break down in the mouth into simple sugars and can be used by the bacteria to cause dental caries are referred to as which of the following?

    a. cariogenic

29. Systemic fluoride can be found in

    c. fluoridated water.

Section VI:
Prevention and Management of Emergencies

This section of the General Chairside portion of the Certified Dental Assisting Examination consists of 12% or 15 questions of the 120 multiple-choice items. The questions related to this section of the General Chairside Dental Assisting Examination are based upon your knowledge of the following:

- Preventing and managing medical emergencies in the dental office
- Preventing and managing a dental emergency

Key Terms

allergy – an overreaction of the body to an allergen
cyanosis – bluish skin tone due to lack of oxygenation
diastolic – bottom reading of a blood pressure
hyperventilation – abnormally rapid and deep breathing resulting in decreased carbon dioxide levels
hypotension – lower-than-normal blood pressure
shock – sudden depression of the vital processes in the body
syncope – fainting
systolic – top reading of a blood pressure

Quick Review Outline

A. Medical Emergencies

   1. The dental assistant must understand the techniques for the prevention of medical emergencies in patients with histories of the following conditions:

      a. AIDS (manifestation of the human immunodeficiency virus)
      b. Alcohol/substance abuse
      c. Allergies
      d. Angina pectoris
      e. Arthritis or rheumatism
      f. Asthma
      g. Blood dyscrasia
      h. Cancer
      i. Cardiovascular disease
      j. Diabetes mellitus or hypoglycemia
      k. Emphysema
      l. Epilepsy
      m. Hepatitis
      n. Hypertension or hypotension
      o. Kidney or liver conditions
      p. Prosthetic joints or heart valve replacement
      q. Respiratory infection
      r. Rheumatic fever or congenital heart disease
      s. Ulcers
      t. Pregnancy

   2. Recognizing medications that are related to the patient's present and/or past medical/dental history is a function of the dental assistant.

   3. You must be able to demonstrate preventive measures to be used following drug administration to avoid drug-induced emergencies.

4. Recognizing the signs and symptoms related to the following specific medical conditions/emergencies likely to occur in the dental office and responding to these emergencies is a responsibility of the dental assistant.

    a. Airway obstruction

    b. Cardiovascular or cerebrovascular accident (stroke)

    c. Diabetic or epileptic related incidents

    d. Reactions to drugs or anesthetics

    e. Respiratory irregularities (hypo or hyperventilation, asthma)

    f. Shock

    g. Syncope (fainting)

    h. Contagious diseases

    i. Allergic reactions

    j. Blood loss

    k. Metabolic or neurologic disease

5. The dental assistant should understand the assembly and maintenance as well as the whereabouts of appropriate emergency supplies, drugs, and equipment.

    a. Recognizing and understanding the uses of drugs in the prevention and/or effective management of an emergency is a function of the dental assistant.

    b. The assistant must know how to assemble the oxygen tank and use it.

    c. The assistant should know basic first aid as it relates to patient care.

    d. If the office has an AED machine, the assistant must know how to use it in the event of cardiac arrest in a patient or coworker.

    e. The assistant should know where the fire extinguisher is and how to use it in the event of a fire.

6. The dental assistant should know how to prepare and post a listing of emergency support personnel in and outside of the office.

B. Dental Emergencies

1. Recognize the signs and symptoms related to specific dental conditions/emergencies likely to occur in the office.

    a. Recognize the types of soft tissue inflammation of the oral cavity.

    b. Identification of contagious oral diseases such as HSV I.

2. Implement and/or assist with appropriate procedure for the management of dental emergencies.

Important Concepts to Know

1. Explain techniques for the prevention of medical emergencies with patients who have a history of medical conditions.
2. Recognize medications that are related to the patient's present and/or past medical/dental history.
3. Demonstrate preventive measures to be used following drug administration to avoid drug-induced emergencies.
4. Recognize the signs and symptoms of specific medical conditions.
5. Respond to the management of chairside emergencies.
6. Demonstrate how to assemble and maintain appropriate emergency supplies, drugs, and equipment.
7. Demonstrate how to prepare and post a listing of emergency support personnel.
8. Explain the procedures for the management of dental emergencies.

Study Checklist

1. Review textbook chapter on medical and dental emergencies.
2. Study terminology related to medical and dental emergencies in the office.
3. Review the American Heart Association's cardiopulmonary resuscitation manual.
4. Review common drugs and medications with both generic and brand names that are used in the treatment of common medical and dental conditions.

Section VI:
Prevention and Management of Emergencies –
Review Questions

Use the Answer Sheet found in Appendix A.

1. Symptoms of heart attack include all the following EXCEPT
   a. profuse sweating.
   b. chest pain.
   c. labored breathing.
   d. erythema.

2. Which of the following is the best prevention of an asthma attack?
   a. bronchodilator
   b. ammonia inhalants
   c. pulse oximeter
   d. automated defibrillator

3. Medical complications for patients diagnosed with AIDS can be prevented by implementing the following procedures:
   a. consulting with patient's physician prior to treatment
   b. postponing dental treatment
   c. minimizing aerosol productions
   d. practicing universal standards (precautions)

4. Signs and symptoms commonly associated with insulin shock (hypoglycemia) include
   a. crushing pain in chest, slurred speech.
   b. cold sweat, weakness, dizziness.
   c. bluish skin tone (cyanosis).
   d. increased rate of respiration/hyperventilation.

5. Which of the following is the recommended method for managing airway obstruction of a foreign body in an adult?
   a. finger sweep to remove object if victim is responsive
   b. abdominal thrusts (Heimlich maneuver)
   c. check for breathing and pulse then begin CPR
   d. place victim in recovery position and administer moderate back blows

6. Acetone breath, dry mouth, thirst, and weak pulse are possible symptoms of
   a. heart attack.
   b. diabetic coma.
   c. hypertension.
   d. epilepsy.

7. Anaphylactic shock is
   a. a chronic allergic reaction.
   b. the result of aspirating a foreign object.
   c. an acute allergic reaction.
   d. best treated with the patient in a seated position.

8. Knowing a patient's medical and dental history might affect
   a. the treatment plan.
   b. the drugs prescribed.
   c. the length of the scheduled appointments.
   d. all of the above.

9. When taking a blood pressure reading, the first sound heard is the
   a. diastolic.
   b. systolic.
   c. carotid pressure.
   d. femoral pressure.

10. Administering a drug in an excess amount is known as
    a. toxemia.
    b. hyperarrested.
    c. actual dose.
    d. overdose.

11. Syncope is also referred to as
    a. hyperventilation.
    b. fainting.
    c. heart failure.
    d. epilepsy.

12. A patient with emphysema may have trouble
    a. focusing.
    b. obtaining a strong pulse.
    c. breathing.
    d. walking.

13. Oftentimes, a patient who has recently had a heart attack will be instructed by their MD to avoid dental treatment for
    a. two weeks.
    b. two months.
    c. six months.
    d. one year.

14. Patients with an autoimmune disorder may sometimes require _____ prior to dental treatment.
    a. an antibiotic prophylactic
    b. a phone call to clear the patient
    c. a complete blood panel
    d. consultation regarding treatment outcomes

15. Patients who are treating alcohol abuse should not be given _____ in the dental office.
    a. antibiotics
    b. mouthwash
    c. fluoride
    d. anesthetics

16. A patient who suffers from angina pectoris routinely carries
    a. nitroglycerine pills.
    b. aspirin.
    c. an inhaler.
    d. Benadryl.

17. Patients who are undergoing cancer treatment may suffer from
    a. dry mouth.
    b. lack of appetite.
    c. increased plaque levels.
    d. all of the above.

18. During the administration of anesthesia, the operator will _____ while delivering anesthetic to avoid injecting directly into an artery.
    a. aspirate
    b. inject quickly
    c. inject slowly
    d. use pressure

19. A patient suddenly becomes disoriented and begins to slur his words. The cause could be
    a. grand mal seizure.
    b. stroke.
    c. heart attack.
    d. respiratory arrest.

20. After receiving anesthesia, the patient informs you that she feels faint and begins to sweat. She indicates she has not had anything to eat that day. You should
    a. give her an ammonia inhalant.
    b. give her orange juice or another high-sugar drink.
    c. prepare to administer CPR.
    d. recline the dental chair into a subsupine position.

21. A proper contact sheet in the event of an emergency should include the
    a. fire department.
    b. ambulance.
    c. police.
    d. all of the above.

22. Emergency supplies should be updated every year to ensure all medications are up to date and have not expired. This is the responsibility of which employee?
    a. dentist
    b. office manager
    c. dental hygienist
    d. backoffice assistant

23. After receiving a local anesthetic, the patient experiences syncope. The best course of action is to
    _____
    a. call 911.
    b. administer oxygen.
    c. lean the patient back in the subsupine position and wait for her to regain consciousness.
    d. administer epinephrine and oxygen and then call 911.

24. Tingling, redness, and mild discomfort before a herpetic lesion presents are collectively called _____
    a. prodromal symptoms.
    b. antipyretic symptoms.
    c. bifurcated symptoms.
    d. none of the above.

25. If a patient begins to have a seizure, the best course of action is to _____
    a. put something between their teeth.
    b. clear an area and let them have the seizure.
    c. call 911 immediately.
    d. administer oxygen.

Section VI:
Prevention and Management of Emergencies –
Answers and Rationales

1. Symptoms of a heart attack incident include all of the following EXCEPT

   d. Erythema means redness of the skin and would not be symptom of a heart attack . All the other symptoms such as profuse sweating, chest pain, and labored breathing are symptoms that can be experienced during a heart attack.

2. Which of the following is the best prevention of an asthma attack?

   a. A bronchodilator would be the best item to use in the event that a patient begins to have an asthma attack. A bronchodilator will open the bronchioles of the lungs and aid the patient in breathing. Ammonia inhalants are used for syncope, a pulse oximeter is a meter used during oral surgery, and a defibrillator would be used to shock the heart into rhythm in the event the patient went into cardiac arrest.

3. Medical complications for patients diagnosed with AIDS can be prevented by implementing the following procedures:

   a. Consulting with the patient's physician prior to treatment is the best way to prevent any kind of medical complication. Patients with AIDS (manifestation of HIV) are very fragile, and their health should be guarded very carefully, so speaking with their physician prior to any treatment will give the dental team vital information. Some physicians require antibiotics or other medical intervention prior to dental treatment. Postponing dental treatment is not necessary if the patient is physically able to tolerate the procedure, and minimizing aerosol and practicing universal precautions is just infection-control practice that the team should be practicing regardless of their patient's health status.

4. Sign and symptoms commonly associated with insulin shock (hypoglycemia) include

   b. Cold sweat, weakness, and dizziness are symptoms associated with insulin shock. The patient should be given a cup of orange juice or some other high-sugar item to help bring their blood sugar level up. Cyanosis, chest pain, slurred speech, and increased respiration are not related to hypoglycemia.

5. Which of the following is the recommended method for managing airway obstruction of a foreign body in a conscious adult?

   b. Abdominal thrusts (Heimlich maneuver) are the best way to dislodge a foreign body airway obstruction. A finger sweep could lodge the item further into the patient's airway, CPR is not indicated for a choking victim *unless* the patient becomes unconscious and the heart stops, and the recovery position is reserved for after the patient has been successfully treated. Back blows are used on infants, not adults.

6. Acetone breath, dry mouth, thirst, and weak pulse are possible symptoms of

   b. Diabetic coma can be characterized by dry mouth, thirst, and weak pulse. These symptoms are not associated with hypertension, epilepsy, or a heart attack.

7. Anaphylactic shock is

   c. An acute allergic reaction is directly related to anaphylactic shock. The onset is sudden and can be characterized with a rash, breathing difficulty, unconsciousness, and eventually death if not treated.

8. Knowing a patient's medical and dental history might affect

   d. all of the above. Knowing a patient's medical and dental history is directly related to the treatment plan you are going to implement, the medications you may prescribe, and the length of the dental appointment. Some patients cannot tolerate certain medications, lengthy appointments where they are required to sit in one position for a long time, or if they are willing to even accept the treatment plan you are offering.

9. When taking a blood pressure reading, the first sound heard is the

   b. Systolic is the reading the appears first and is the top number. This number represents the force exerted on the arteries when the heart contracts.

10. Administering a drug in an excess amount is known as

    d. An overdose is exactly what it states: an overadministration of medication. If an overdose is not addressed, death may result.

11. Syncope is also referred to as

    b. Fainting is another name for syncope.

12. A patient with emphysema may have trouble in

    c. Breathing is a common problem with patients who have emphysema. Patients who have emphysema have compromised lung function and most often find it hard to breathe.

13. Oftentimes, a patient who has recently had a heart attack will be instructed by their MD to avoid dental treatment for

    c. Six months is the standard amount of time that a physician recommends that a patient wait until dental treatment is performed.

14. Patients with an autoimmune disorder may sometimes require _____ prior to dental treatment.

    a. An antibiotic prophylactic due to the nature of the patient who has a compromised immune system. Oftentimes, the patient's MD will require an antibiotic prescription for the patient prior to dental treatment.

15. Patients who are treating alcohol abuse should not be given _____ in dental office.

    b. Mouthwash often contains alcohol, so giving patients alcohol may interfere with medications that the patient is taking to combat the addiction.

16. A patient who suffers from angina pectoris routinely carries

    a. Nitroglycerine pills are taken sublingually when chest pain is experienced to alleviate pain and discomfort. Aspirin, inhalers, and Benadryl are not used when treating angina.

17. Patients who are undergoing cancer treatment may suffer from

    d. All of the above are symptoms that a patient may be experiencing while undergoing cancer treatment.

18. During the administration of anesthesia, the operator will _____ while delivering anesthetic to avoid injecting directly into an artery.

    a. aspirate – Aspirating (pulling the plunger back on the syringe) to check for blood will ensure that the operator is not injecting directly into the artery, which can cause a flushed feeling with heart palpitations.

19. A patient suddenly becomes disoriented and begins to slur his words. The cause could be

    b. A stroke can cause immediate disorientation, slurring of speech, and sometimes numbness on one side of the body.

20. After receiving anesthesia, the patient informs you that she feels faint and begins to sweat. She indicates she has not had anything to eat that day. You should

    b. give her orange juice or another high-sugar drink, because chances are her blood sugar level has dropped and is causing hypoglycemic symptoms.

21. A proper contact sheet in the event of an emergency should include the

    d. All of the above should be included on your emergency contact sheet. This sheet should be displayed in an area where everyone can see it.

22. Emergency supplies should be updated every year to ensure all medications are not expired. This is the responsibility of which employee?

    d. Generally, the backoffice assistant manages all the emergency equipment and its maintenance. Sometimes there will be a designated safety officer, but most often that person is also the backoffice assistant.

23. After receiving a local anesthesia, the patient experiences syncope. The best course of action is to _____.

    c. Lean the patient back in the subsupine position and wait for her to regain consciousness. Once blood returns to the brain, the patient should respond within seconds. If the patient stays unconscious for more than 2 minutes, maintain their airway, call 911, and monitor their breathing and pulse.

24. Tingling, redness, and mild discomfort before a herpetic lesion presents are collectively called _____.

    a. Prodromal symptoms are any symptoms that present prior to the disease manifesting itself into a raised lesion. For example, a scratchy throat and fatigue are prodromal symptoms that occur before the flu. A tingling lip or pain below the surface of the tissue is a prodromal symptom that occurs prior to a herpetic breakout.

25. If a patient begins to have a grand mal seizure, the best course of action is _____.

    b. Clear an area and let the patient have the seizure. Do not place anything in between the patient's teeth or administer any medications or oxygen. After the patient has the seizure, place him or her in the recovery position and allow the patient to rest. Calling 911 usually isn't necessary unless the patient was injured during the seizure and needs medical attention.

Section VII:
Office Operations

This topic of the General Chairside portion of the Certified Dental Assisting Examination consists of 10% or 12 questions of the 120 multiple-choice items. Testing topics and objectives are outlined below for this portion of the exam. The questions related to this section of the general chairside assisting exam are based upon your knowledge of the following:

- Supply and inventory control
- Maintenance of equipment/instruments
- Patient reception, communication, and accounting
- Legal aspects and responsibilities of dentistry

Key Terms

inventory control system – a method to track supplies in the office

malpractice – incorrect or negligent treatment given to a patient by a doctor, dentist, or health care provider

OSHA – regulating body that enforces the requirements established for employers to protect their employees

Patient record – legal documentation of a patient's care and treatments

State Dental Practice Act – state regulations that describe legal restrictions and controls on the dentist, the hygienist, and dental assistants

Quick Review Outline

A. Supply and Inventory Control
  1. Maintaining and controlling supply levels is an ongoing duty.
     a. Recording and keeping an accurate inventory of items used and needed is an important function of the dental assistant. Having adequate supplies of inventory keeps the office running smoothly.
     b. Implementing a system of ordering supplies, instruments, and equipment to maintain specified levels is vital in maintaining office production. There are several methods of inventory control, which include manual card systems, computer autoship, and the grocery list method, which just means that you keep a running list, and when consumables become low, you make a note and then order at regular intervals.
     c. Rotating expendable supplies according to the **inventory control system** takes advantage of keeping adequate amounts of inventory on hand, which gives you lead time when replenishing stock.
     d. The management of backorders according to the inventory control system aids the office in scheduling and performing procedures when there is adequate supply on hand. Scheduling future treatment while having an idea of when backordered supplies will arrive is ideal.
     e. rotate nonexpendables
  2. Maintain security and records of controlled substances.

B. Maintenance of Equipment/Instruments
  1. The dental assistant must understand the importance of performing scheduled preventive maintenance on the equipment and instruments in the dental operatory as per manufacturers' instructions. Maintaining dental equipment is part of the assistant's responsibility. Some of the maintenance that may be required could include:
     a. cleaning and inspecting the autoclave
     b. cleaning and inspecting the ultrasonic
     c. cleaning the automatic film processor and replenishing/changing solutions
     d. changing the debris traps and running the evacuation system on a daily basis
     e. Maintaining handpieces by inspecting and regular cleaning, lubricating, and sterilization is a daily responsibility of the assistant.

f. Maintaining the nitrous oxide/oxygen tanks and equipment that is related to their use should be done on a regular basis for both safety and efficacy.

g. The dental assistant is responsible for updating and replenishing the medical emergencies kit. Checking expiration dates and level of emergency supplies is key when it comes to safety for the patient in the dental office.

h. The dental assistant must ensure the sharpness and effectiveness of hand instruments. New instruments should be ordered when needed. This helps the operator do their job to the best of their abilities.

i. The assistant must order durable goods as needed.

2. The dental assistant should provide appropriate care and storage of supplies such as sterile disposable products, nitrous oxide, and oxygen.

C. Patient Reception, Communication, and Accounting

1. Communicating effectively and establishing good working relationships with patients and with other members of the dental care team is an essential part of being a productive member. You should be able to communicate with your coworkers effectively when it comes to patient care.

2. Seating and dismissing patients is a responsibility of the backoffice assistant. Making sure that patients are greeted and their families are made welcome is an important part of internal marketing and patient care. Upon dismissal, it is important that the patient leaves without unanswered questions, in good condition, and knowledgeable of the treatment that was performed. Follow-up appointments, if needed, should be discussed before the patient leaves the treatment room.

3. The assistant should become familiar with the appointment-control process. Scheduling treatment and the proper amount of time for each of those procedures ensures that the office runs smoothly and patients are not kept waiting. Buffer periods and adequate lunch breaks should be observed.

4. The assistant should feel comfortable and be knowledgeable about explaining fees charged to a patient as directed by the dentist.

5. It is important to know and understand basic concepts of third-party payment such as the various types of insurance payments.

6. When appropriate and after consulting with the dentist, the assistant should feel comfortable initiating a referral procedure for the patient. Referring patients to a specialist should be an activity that is natural to the office. There is no office that can perform with proficiency every dental procedure available. At one time or another, a patient must be referred out for treatment that is beyond the skill level of the office.

7. With advances in technology, everyone in the office should be familiar with computers and dental software and be able to use them with ease in the dental office.

8. Financial management of the dental office

D. Legal Aspects of Dentistry

1. Patient Records

a. It is imperative that the assistant be able to understand and identify the legal significance of medical and dental histories. Accurate and regularly updated health histories protect both the patient and the office. It is the responsibility of the assistant to update the patient's medical history at regular intervals.

b. The assistant should be able to identify items included as part of a legally documented **patient record**. It is important for the assistant to be able to list medications, history of illness, past surgery, refusal of recommended treatment, and past dental work that was performed at another office. These and other items could be of legal interest later on.

c. Offices sometimes lend radiographs or other treatment records to other offices when sharing patients. It is important to implement precautions such as not releasing any personal financial information and requiring the patient to sign a release to send dental treatment records out. This is important to keep in mind when lending records to another dental office.

d. There are two parts of the dental chart. The first part is the treatment and second is the financial. Normally, financial portions of the chart are not sent out to other offices. Only the treatment records, which include treatment notes, radiographs, and other diagnostic information, are shared. You must be able to differentiate among the various types of patient data in the dental office.

e. When filing items, including radiographs, medical/dental histories, correspondence, insurance forms, etc., into individual patient records, it is important that treatment information is stored in the treatment portion of the chart and financial information is kept in a separate financial area.

f. When recording patient telephone communication, the date, time, information discussed, and who you spoke with should be noted in the chart. All consultation information, both medical and dental, should be documented by issuing the patient a treatment plan and notes regarding discussion of the needs of the patient. Any consultation with the patient's medical doctor should be noted with a follow-up letter from the physician, if possible. This is a legal issue and should not be overlooked.

2. Legal Responsibilities and Regulations

a. The factors and precautions necessary to prevent lawsuits against dental personnel include recording all treatment, taking an accurate medical history, and providing full disclosure to the patient before and after treatment. This means providing a treatment plan signed by the patient and a consent form, which is also signed by the patient.

b. Identifying the responsibilities and/or obligations of the dentist and patients in the dentist–patient relationship includes getting honesty from the patient as well as compliance with all recommendations by the dentist.

c. Obtaining consent for routine and emergency office dental care is very important for both legal and financial reasons. The patient must know ahead of time what treatment needs to be performed and how they are expected to meet the financial obligation. Even though it is an emergency, full disclosure and understanding must be implied, and the patient must consent by signing a treatment plan.

d. Maintaining the patient's rights to privacy according to the Health Insurance Portability and Accountability Act (HIPAA) regulations is imperative, as the HIPAA privacy laws are federally mandated. The dentist or any team member is forbidden by law to disclose patient personal information to anyone, including family members or outside entities. The patient must be informed in writing and the HIPAA form signed and maintained in the patient's permanent record.

e. Identifying the actions that a dental assistant should take after a threat to sue for **malpractice** by a patient would include contacting an attorney and not speaking to anyone regarding the case. The attorney will direct you in all actions.

f. Recognizing the legal responsibilities of the dental assistant in relation to the **State Dental Practice Act** requires a thorough knowledge of what your individual state allows you to do under your particular license. Ignorance of the law is no excuse for performing a procedure you are not legally allowed to perform. You are still at risk for liability. Performing procedures that are illegal just because your employer tells you to do so doesn't make you immune to a lawsuit. Know your permitted duties and never deviate from them, no matter what you are told by another.

g. Documentation of any patient refusal of recommended routine and emergency treatment is required. If a patient refuses radiographs, periodontal treatment, or any other restorative procedure and in the future suffers irreparable harm because they did not take the recommendation of the office, you could be subjected to a lawsuit. It is important to have documentation that indicates you recommended intervention to give you leverage in the event of a lawsuit.

h. Be aware of updates in **Occupational Safety and Health Administration (OSHA)** and Centers for Disease Control and Prevention (CDC) guidelines. Maintaining office compliance is important because offices are both federally and state regulated. They must follow rules and guidelines for the safety of both the patient and the dental team. These laws, regulations, and guidelines can be enforced by outside entities that may impose fines if they are not followed. It is imperative that the office stay current on updates and current guidelines for both safety and legal purposes.

Important Concepts to Know

1. Understand supply and inventory in the dental office.
2. Explain the importance of securing and maintaining inventory of controlled substances.
3. Understand the proper maintenance of equipment and instruments.
4. Demonstrate proper practices related to patient reception, communication, and accounting practices in the dental office.
5. Understand completely the legal aspects of dentistry.
6. Understand current CDC and OSHA laws and regulations.

Study Checklist

1. Review terminology as it relates to office operations.
2. Read textbook chapter on the legal aspects of dentistry.
3. Review skills for patient reception and communication.
4. Review sections in your text on OSHA and SDS maintenance.
5. Review chapter sections as they relate to dental insurance and patient accounting.
6. Research and study current CDC and OSHA guidelines for the dental field.

Section VII:
Office Operations – Review Questions

Use the Answer Sheet found in Appendix A.

1. Your supervising dentist asks you to perform a function you are not legally permitted to do even though he/she tells you they will take responsibility. Would it be appropriate to perform the function?
   a. Only if he/she watches you
   b. Only if the patient consents to it
   c. Only if there is nobody else to do it
   d. It is never all right to perform functions outside of your legally permitted duties.

2. _____ supervision means that the dentist is in the office or treatment facility and personally authorizes treatment to be performed.
   a. Direct
   b. Indirect
   c. General
   d. Personal

3. Malpractice is considered
   a. a misdemeanor.
   b. performing an act that a "reasonable and prudent person would perform."
   c. unethical conduct.
   d. professional negligence.

4. _____ is the science dealing with the law as it applies to dentistry.
   a. Dental jurisprudence
   b. Ethics.
   c. Malpractice.
   d. *Respondeat superior*

5. When a patient breaks an appointment, this may be interpreted as
   a. abandonment.
   b. contributory negligence.
   c. forgetfulness.
   d. malpractice.

6. In each state, the _____ contains the legal restrictions and controls that govern the practice of dentistry.
   a. ADA code of ethics
   b. federal principles of ethics
   c. State Board of Dentistry
   d. State Dental Practice Act

7. Failure to comply with the Dental Practice Act or any other laws governing the practice of dentistry could result in
   a. a fine.
   b. license revocation.
   c. a and b
   d. none of the above.

8. The area on the daily schedule that is set aside for emergencies is called a _____
   a. buffer period.
   b. static time.
   c. lunch hour.
   d. interim time.

9. _____ ensure that a practice has a constant supply of materials and eliminates the need to store an abundance of one item.
   a. Automatic shipments
   b. Bulk ordering
   c. Purchase quantity
   d. Limited ordering

10. Accounts payable are
    a. money that is leaving the practice.
    b. supplies purchased for the office.
    c. fixed overhead expenses.
    d. insurance payments.

11. If a team member discloses a patient's personal information to any unauthorized person, this is a direct violation of the
    a. code of ethics.
    b. HIPAA law.
    c. dental malpractice act.
    d. dental jurisprudence regulations.

12. Which of the following would not be part of the treatment record?
    a. notes from previous restorative treatment
    b. recent periodontal probe readings
    c. EOB sheet sent by the insurance company
    d. radiographs

13. The best way to extend the life of your handpieces is to
    a. properly clean, inspect, sterilize, and lubricate after each use.
    b. call the repairman to service the handpiece every six months.
    c. rely on the dentist to perform the maintenance when needed.
    d. purchase a warranty for each of the handpieces.

14. If a patient refuses full-mouth radiographs when due, the assistant should do the following:
    a. Let the patient know that radiographs have low exposure and remind them of the shielding equipment that you will be using.
    b. Explain that the dentist needs them to do a complete diagnosis.
    c. Remind the patient they may be excused from the practice.
    d. all of the above

15. Which laws determine what the dental assistant is legally able to perform?
    a. federal laws
    b. state laws
    c. township mandates
    d. the dentist he/she is employed by

16. Each state has legal restrictions and controls on dental professionals and the practice of dentistry. The restrictions are collectively referred to as what?
    a. ADAA code of ethics
    b. State Board of Dentistry restrictions
    c. State Dental Practice Act
    d. State Dental Ethics Accountability Act

17. What does HIPAA stand for?
    a. Health Insurance Portability and Accountability Act
    b. Health Insurance Privacy and Accountability Act
    c. Health Institute of Public and Accountability
    d. Hospital Internal Protocol Practice Act

18. Which answer below does NOT apply to confidentiality?
    a. the patient has a right to privacy
    b. the dental office does not disclose personal information about the patient
    c. the patient can talk to their insurance company about treatment
    d. the patient must give written permission to have information released to others

19. Which portion of the chart is not included in the patient's clinical record?
    a. financial
    b. treatment that needs to be completed
    c. health history
    d. periodontal charting

20. When presenting a treatment plan, when should the patient be told about all the risk, benefits, and treatment options?
    a. after they sign the pretreatment plan
    b. before they sign the pretreatment plan
    c. throughout the examination
    d. after treatment has been completed

21. During a malpractice court case, which of the following may apply in regard to dental records?
    a. They are always written in pencil.
    b. They are never admissible in court due to privacy issues.
    c. They always are sent to the patient for review prior to the trial date.
    d. They are used in court as legal evidence.

22. Legal restrictions that control the actions of the dentist and staff would be found in
    a. a JADA journal
    b. an ADA journal
    c. the State Dental Practice Act
    d. an "implied consent" form

23. Malpractice is the same as
    a. professional negligence.
    b. failure to exercise due care.
    c. an act of commission.
    d. all of the above.

Section VII:
Office Operations – Answers and Rationales

1. Your supervising dentist asks you to perform a function you are not legally permitted to do. Would it be appropriate to perform the function?

   d. It is never all right for you to perform a function outside of your permitted duties, no matter what your employer says they will do. It is ultimately your license that will be in jeopardy. You can be fined and/or lose your license, which means that you will lose your livelihood.

2. _____ supervision means that the dentist is in the office or treatment facility and personally authorizes treatment to be performed.

   a. Direct

3. Malpractice is considered

   d. Professional negligence is considered the same as malpractice in that the welfare and well-being of the patient were compromised during the delivery of dental treatment.

4. _____ is the science dealing with the law as it applies to dentistry.

   a. Dental jurisprudence is the term used to include statues regulating the legal aspects of the practice of dentistry.

5. When a patient breaks an appointment, this may be interpreted as

   b. Contributory negligence is based on the philosophy that the patient should be involved in the overall delivery of dental treatment. By scheduling and attending the appointment, the patient is actively participating in the delivery of care. When a patient breaks an appointment, the patient is contributing to the breakdown in care.

6. In each state, the _____ contains the legal restrictions and controls that govern the practice of dentistry.

   d. State Dental Practice Act regulates the laws that all dental professionals are required to practice under. When in violation and a complaint is filed, the dental professional can be investigated by the Board of Dental Examiners for their state, and the Board has the right to file suit on behalf of the victim.

7. Failure to comply with the Dental Practice Act or any other laws governing the practice of dentistry could result in

   c. a and b – A dental professional can be fined and/or lose their license if they fail to comply with the Dental Practice Act.

8. The area on the daily schedule that is set aside for emergencies is called

   a. buffer period – A buffer period can be for anything. It is just a block of time set aside for an activity. It could be emergencies, staff meetings, or just a short period of time to catch up and get back on schedule.

9. _____ ensure that a practice has a constant supply of materials and eliminates the need to store an abundance of one item.

   a. Automatic shipments – This form of supply ordering sends a certain type of supply such as toothbrushes on a regular interval. This saves on storage space and constant monitoring.

10. Accounts payable are

    a. money that is leaving the practice – Any money that is paid out for supplies, equipment, rent, or any other expenses can be considered accounts payable.

11. If a team member discloses a patient's personal information to any unauthorized person, this is a direct violation of the

    b. HIPAA law – This is a federal law that prohibits the discussion of personal medical treatment of any kind with any unauthorized person. An authorized person would include someone that the patient has specifically designated in writing.

12. Which of the following would not be part of the treatment record?

    c. EOB sheet sent by the insurance company is not part of the treatment record. Probe readings, radiographs, and treatment notes are all part of the treatment record. The EOB is part of the financial record.

13. The best way to extend the life of your handpieces is to

    a. properly clean, inspect, sterilize, and lubricate after each use – It is the responsibility of the assistant to maintain the equipment in the office, with the exception of repairing it. Most equipment, if maintained properly, can last years without being repaired.

14. If a patient refuses full-mouth radiographs when due, the assistant should do the following:

    d. **All of the above – The patient must be reminded of all of the safety precautions that are implemented when taking radiographs, they must also know that the dentist cannot make an effective diagnosis without them, and they may be excused from the practice. Asking the patient to sign a refusal is not adequate. This tactic will not work if you are sued, because having the patient sign a refusal and continuing to perform treatment is nothing more than consensual negligence. You both know they require radiographs and you both continue with treatment.**

15. Which laws determine what the dental assistant is legally able to perform?

    b. **state laws – State laws mandate what dental assistant are legally able to perform. Each state has its own standards and laws. When laws are broken, the state's attorney would file charges and take action on behalf of the plaintiff or victim.**

16. Each state has legal restrictions and controls on dental professionals and the practice of dentistry. The restrictions are collectively referred to as what?

    c. **State Dental Practice Act – Each state has its own State Dental Practice Act that mandates legally what dental professionals are legally able to perform and licensure required to perform those duties.**

17. What does HIPAA stand for?

    a. **Health Insurance Portability and Accountability Act – This act protects the privacy of individually identifiable health information. The HIPAA Security Rule sets national standards for the security of electronic protected health information. The confidentiality provisions of the Patient Safety Rule protect identifiable information being used to improve patient safety.**

18. Which answer below does NOT apply to confidentiality?

    c. **The patient can talk to their insurance company about treatment – The patient can talk to their insurance company and, in some instances, file a grievance against the dental office with their insurance company at any time. Confidentiality does not apply to this situation.**

19. Which portion of the chart is not included in the patient's clinical record?

    a. **financial – The financial portion is kept separate from the clinical record. Financial records reflect payments, credits, and insurance information, and the clinical record shows treatment plans, procedure notes, and items related to direct care of the patient.**

20. When presenting a treatment plan, when should the patient be told about all the risk, benefits, and treatment options?

    b. **before they sign the pretreatment plan – Before signing any treatment plan, the patient should have an understanding of what it is they are signing and assigning all the risk and benefits to treatment.**

21. During a malpractice court case, which of the following may apply in regard to dental records?

    d. **They are used in court as legal evidence. – Dental records are legal documents, so it is imperative for you to list any and everything possible in the event there is a lawsuit filed.**

22. Legal restrictions that control the actions of the dentist and staff would be found in

    c. **the State Dental Practice Act.**

23. Malpractice is the same as

    a. **professional negligence.**

CHAPTER 2 – RADIATION HEALTH AND SAFETY

The Radiation Health and Safety (RHS) exam consists of 100 questions, all of which are multiple choice. There are four content areas of focus in this component of the Dental Assisting National Board Examination. These content areas are:

- Expose and Evaluate (26% or 26 questions)
  - Properly assess patients to determine proper radiation techniques and prepare the equipment to use
  - Describe how to properly acquire radiographic images
  - Effectively evaluate radiographic images for diagnostic value
  - Explain how to manage patients before, during, and after radiographic exposures
- Quality Assurance and Radiology Regulations (21% or 21 questions)
  - Evaluate and maintain quality of radiographic supplies and equipment and correct errors in exposure
  - Describe and implement proper regulations related to storage and disposal of chemicals related to radiography as well as proper methods of duplication and transfer of radiographs
- Radiation Safety for Patients and Operators (31% or 31 questions)
  - Identify ADA guidelines for frequency of exposure
  - Apply principles of radiation protection
  - Demonstrate proper techniques to protect patients from exposure to radiation
  - Address patient concerns related to radiation exposure, including acquisition of consent or refusal
  - Demonstrate proper techniques for maintaining the safety of the operator while exposing radiographic images
  - Describe techniques for monitoring individual exposure to radiation
- Infection Control (22% or 22 questions)
  - Demonstrate use of standard precautions for radiographic equipment
  - Demonstrate implementation of standard precautions for patients and the operator during radiographic procedures

This chapter provides an outline and review of the testing topics and objectives on the Radiation Health and Safety component of the DANB exam. It is anticipated that this component of the examination will take 1 hour and 15 minutes to complete.

Section I: Expose and Evaluate

This section of the Radiation Health and Safety component of the Certified Dental Assisting Examination consists of 26% or 26 of the 100 multiple-choice items. The questions related to this section of the examination are based upon your knowledge of the following.

- Assessment and preparation of the proper radiographic technique and equipment to be used
- Acquisition of radiographic images of proper diagnostic quality
- Evaluation of radiographic images for proper diagnostic quality
- Patient management before, during, and after exposure

Key Terms

developer – the first chemical solution used to process radiographs

enamel – tooth structure that covers the outside of the crown of the tooth; the hardest living tissue in the body

fixer – the second chemical solution used in processing radiographs

identification dot – a raised dot on the x-ray film to facilitate the mounting process

latent image – image formed by crystal halide that is exposed to radiation; the image doesn't form until it has been exposed to chemicals for a specified period of time

maxillary sinus – forms a large cavity above the roots of the maxillary molars

radiolucent – black region on the x-ray indicating where radiation passed through the tissue

radiopaque – white or light region on the x-ray indicating where radiation was blocked by tissue or a substance

replenish – to refill or fill with new solutions

sinus – air-filled cavity in the skull in and around the nasal region

supernumerary teeth – extra teeth; usually dwarfed in size or shape

Quick Review Outline

I. Expose and Evaluate

    A. The dental assistant should be able to demonstrate patient assessment, determine the proper technique, and prepare the equipment based upon the technique being used.

        1. Describe patient preparation for radiographic exposures.

            a. Prior to exposure of radiographs, inspect the head and neck for any reasons radiographs cannot be taken such as physical disability or malformations.

            b. Identify removable appliances or foreign objects such as earrings, tongue rings, partials, dentures, retainers, or any other metal items that may create an artifact on the radiograph.

        2. Select the appropriate radiographic technique.

            a. Identify the use and purpose of various intraoral and extraoral radiographs. x-ray machines are commonly used safely and effectively in dentistry. They are used when fast, highly penetrating images are needed. They are used for diagnosing decay and various cancers, during orthodontic treatment, to evaluate areas of interest prior to dental surgery, and for general dental procedures.

                i. periapical radiographs – radiographs that capture the crown of the tooth as well as the entire root and surrounding structures (Figure 2-1A).

                ii. bitewing radiographs – radiographs that capture the first 1/3 of the tooth. This radiograph does not include the root or apex of the tooth (Figure 2-1B).

                iii. occlusal radiographs – This film is placed along the occlusal plane and shows the surrounding maxillary or mandibular bone structures, occlusal surfaces, and crowns of the teeth (Figure 2-1C).

                iv. panoramic radiograph – This radiograph utilizes a special panoramic x-ray unit which rotates around the patient's head, capturing the entire maxilla, mandible, and surrounding structures on one film. The patient stays stationary while the unit moves around the patient's head (Figure 2-1D).

                v. cephalometric radiographs – lateral and posteroanterior extraoral head films (Figure 2-1E). These radiographs are generally used for orthodontic and/or surgical cases.

                vi. Other extraoral radiographs may be used when patients cannot or will not open their mouth. Disabled patients or patients with trismus or temporomandibular joint disorders may not be able to tolerate the placement of intraoral films, so alternate extraoral film techniques are used.

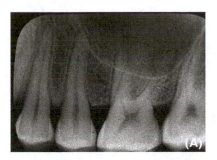
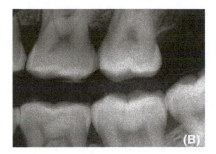
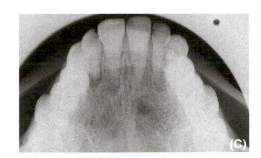
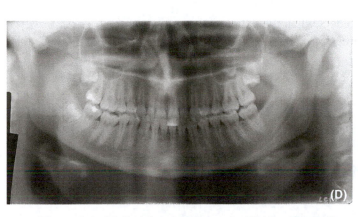
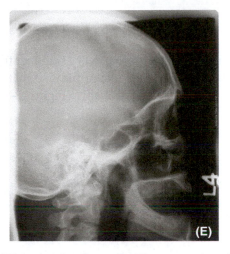

Figure 2-1 (A) Peripheral radiograph, (B) bite-wing radiograph, (C) occlusal radiograph, (D) panoramic radiograph, and (E) cephalometric radiograph

b. The dental assistant should be able to select appropriate radiographic film to examine, view, or survey conditions, teeth, or landmarks. The following are some of the most common.

    i. caries

    ii. temporomandibular joint

    iii. periodontal conditions

    iv. apical pathology such as abscesses

    v. sinus areas

    vi. dental anomalies, such as **supernumerary teeth**, tori, resorption, and ankylosis

    vii. edentulous arches

    viii. localization of impacted teeth, foreign objects, etc.

    ix. dental implants

c. Describe technique modifications based upon anatomical variations.

    i. Patients with a high gag reflex may benefit from topical spray.

    ii. Patients with a shallow palate or floor of the mouth may need a smaller film size or sensor.

    iii. Patients with a smaller oral cavity may not be able to use the Rinn film holders.

3. Select appropriate equipment for radiographic techniques

    a. The dental assistant should be able to select appropriate equipment for radiographic techniques and be able to describe the purpose or advantage of accessories for radiographic techniques, including film holders, cotton rolls, bitewing tabs, bite blocks, lead apron, and thyroid collar.

        i. Film-holding devices (such as Snap-A-Ray or Rinn) align the x-ray beam with the film in the patient's mouth. These devices stabilize the film in the mouth and reduce the need to re-expose the patient to additional radiation (Figure 2-2 A and B).

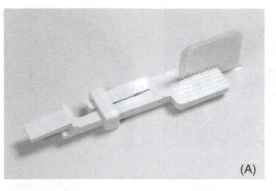 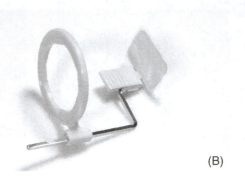

(A) (B)

Figure 2-2 (A) Snap-A-Ray and (B) Rinn XCP

   ii. Cotton rolls are used to stabilize film holders when the patient has missing teeth.

  iii. Bitewing tabs secure films so that the areas of interest on both the maxillary and mandibular arch are represented evenly (Figure 2-3).

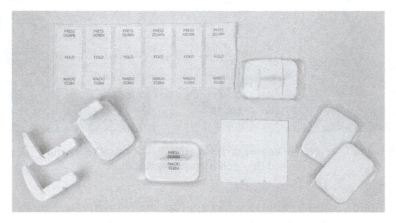

Figure 2-3 Bite-wing loops and tabs

   iv. Bite blocks aid in the stabilization of radiographs during exposure when individual exposures are needed.

   v. The lead apron with thyroid collar is used to protect the patient's chest, reproductive, and thyroid areas from secondary or scatter radiation

b. The dental assistant should be able to identify and select the appropriate image receptor size and film speed (sensitivity) depending on patient characteristics and exposure technique indicated (Table 2-1).

Table 2-1: Intraoral Film Sizes and Uses

Film Size	Description/Use
No. 0	Child size
No. 1	Narrow anterior film size
No. 2	Adult size
No. 3	Long bitewing films size
No. 4	Occlusal film size

   i. You may see speed groups such as super, ultra, or ekta. Although these names tell you little or nothing about the actual film speed, the American National Standards Institute (ANSI) uses letters of the alphabet to assign film speed.

   ii. Speed group "A" is considered the lowest, with "F" as the fastest. Currently, only K-speed and E-speed films are used for dental radiographs.

iii. Factors that determine film speed or sensitivity refer to the amount of radiation required to produce a radiograph in dentistry. The faster the film speed, the less radiation is required to get an acceptable dental radiograph.

iv. Halide crystals embedded in the emulsion on the film affect the speed or sensitivity of the film. The larger the crystals the faster the film and less radiation exposure the film requires to produce an image. However, the larger the crystals the less distinction and sharpness the film produces.

c. The dental assistant should be able to describe the purpose of various film packets.

   i. Periapical film used to examine the entire tooth and its surrounding structures.

      a. Size 0: 35 × 22 mm anterior, posterior, children

      b. Size 1: 40 × 22 mm anterior, posterior, adult (standard size)

      c. Size 2: 40.5 × 30.5 mm posterior, adult (all posterior)

   ii. Bitewing film used for the examining interproximal surfaces

      a. Size 0: 35 × 22 mm (anterior, posterior)

      b. Size 2: 40.5 × 30.5 mm (posterior)

      c. Size 3: 54 × 27 mm (posterior)

   iii. Occlusal films

      a. Size 4: 57 × 76 mm occlusal (captures either maxillary or mandibular arch)

   iv. Panoramic Film

      a. 5 × 12 inches (captures both dental arches, sinus, nasal bones, and lower orbits of the eyes)

   v. Cephalometric Film

      a. 5 × 7 inches or 8 × 10 inches (captures a side view of the entire skull to include the first four to five vertebrae)

   vi. Double film packets are individual film packets that contain two films. These are primarily used when an additional duplicate film of a particular area needs to be exposed. Such occasions may be when one film stays with the patient record and the other would go to either a referral or the insurance company. The State of California has passed a law that states the dental office must provide the patient a copy of their complete patient records. Duplicate radiographs have become more common in these offices.

B. The dental assistant should be able to demonstrate acquisition of radiographs using proper imaging techniques for both traditional and digital radiography.

  1. Describe how to acquire radiographic images using various techniques

    a. The dental assistant should be able to define the following radiographic exposure concepts.

      i. film speed – This refers to the amount of radiation required to produce a radiograph of standard density. The faster the film speed, the less radiation required to get a standard density radiograph.

      ii. kilovolt – (kV) a unit of electromotive force, equal to 1000 volts. High kilovoltage is essential for the production of dental x-rays.

      iii. milliampere – (mA) the milliampere is one thousandth of an ampere. In radiography, the milliamperage determines the number of electrons available at the filament.

      iv. collimation – the restriction of the useful beam to an appropriate size; generally, to a diameter of 2¾ in. (7 cm) at the skin surface

      v. filtration – the use of absorbers for selectively absorbing or screening out the low-energy x-rays from the primary beam

      vi. film density – the degree to which a processed film is darkened

      vii. **latent images** – the invisible image produced when the film is exposed to the x-ray

    b. The dental assistant should demonstrate proper techniques during intraoral radiographic exposures

      i. The dental assistant should be able to define the factors that influence the quality of a radiographic exposure.

a. mA setting determines the density of the exposure. Increasing the mA will darken the image, and decreasing the mA will lighten the image.

b. kVp setting will determine the contrast of the image, giving the image varying degrees of darkness and opacity.

c. Primary beam angles (horizontal and vertical) will change the image's length. Therefore, when the primary beam has too much vertical angulation, the image can be foreshortened or elongated. If the primary beam has too much horizontal angulation, the individual items in the exposure can be overlapped onto each other, decreasing accurateness, especially interproximally.

d. PID (cone) length will determine the sharpness of an image. Using a shorter cone will give you a sharper image, whereas using a longer cone or placing the PID far away from the area of interest will cause the image to appear blurry.

e. Exposure time can determine whether an exposure has correct contrast. An image that is underexposed will appear too light, and an exposure that is overexposed will appear very dark.

ii. The dental assistant should be able to compare paralleling and bisecting angle techniques, including their advantages and disadvantages.

a. The differences between paralleling and bisecting techniques include the distances used, the angle the assistant selects, and the film-holding method (either using a film holder or the patient using their finger).

b. Paralleling technique occurs when the film packet is parallel to the teeth while the central beam of radiation is toward the teeth (Figure 2-4).

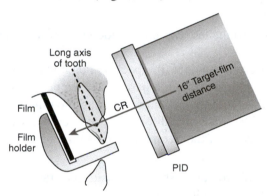

Figure 2-4 Paralleling technique

c. Bisecting technique occurs when the central rays are aimed perpendicularly to the bisector (the imaginary line that bisects the angle formed by the film and tooth) and therefore do not actually strike either the tooth or the film at a right angle (Figure 2-5).

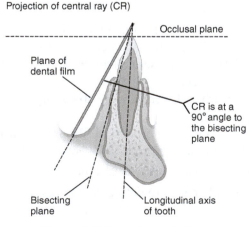

Figure 2-5 Bisecting technique

iii. The dental assistant should be able to name the parts and functions of a radiograph film packet (Figure 2-6A and B) as well as the parts of a digital sensor.

   a. black paper that surrounds film, which aids in excluding any light

   b. Lead foil is used to absorb some of the radiation that passes through the film and helps prevent scatter of radiation to the surrounding tissue.

   c. plastic waterproof and lightproof outer covering

   d. digital film sensor

   e. digital sensor cord

   f. digital USB connector

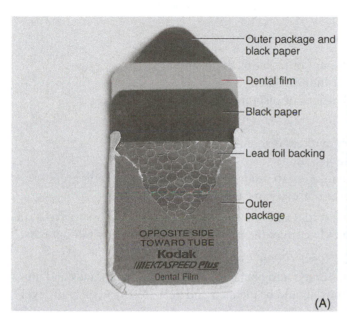

Outer package and black paper

Dental film

Black paper

Lead foil backing

Outer package

OPPOSITE SIDE TOWARD TUBE
Kodak
IIIEKTASPEED Plus
Dental Film

(A)

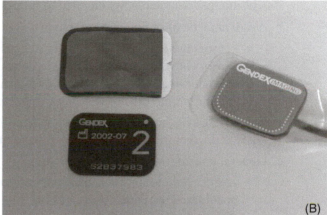

(B)

Figure 2-6 (A) Film packet (B) digital sensor

c. The dental assistant should demonstrate proper techniques during extraoral radiographic exposures.

   i. The dental assistant should be able to identify the function and maintenance of film cassettes and intensifying screens.

      a. Film cassettes hold and protect the film. Most cassettes are rigid and flat, but panoramic radiographs use rigid or flexible, flat, or curved cassettes. These cassettes must be cleaned with a soft cloth and maintained, as any cassette that is damaged can introduce light leaks that will cause film to fog.

      b. Intensifying screen will transfer x-ray energy into visible light. The visible light exposes the screen film. These intensifying screens reduce the radiation required to expose the film so that the patient is exposed to less radiation during the radiography process. These screens must be cleaned with a soft cloth and must not be scratched, as these screens are coated with fluorescent crystals that are required for the screen to intensify the film that is being exposed.

   ii. The dental assistant should be able to describe the appropriate technique for patient positioning during radiographic exposure.

      a. *Panoramic radiography*, also called *panoramic x-ray*, is a two-dimensional (2-D) *dental x-ray* examination that captures the entire mouth in a single image, including the teeth, upper and lower jaws, and surrounding structures and tissues. Generally, the patient stands upright while the film canister travels around the patient's head to produce the image.

      b. A cephalometric x-ray is an extraoral radiograph that enables the orthodontist to capture a complete radiographic image of the side of the face. Cephalometric x-rays are extraoral, meaning that no plates or film are inserted inside the mouth. Cephalometric x-rays display the nasal and sinus passages and bones of the face and cranium, which are missed by intraoral bitewing x-rays.

    iii. The dental assistant should demonstrate a basic understanding of cone-beam computed tomography (CBCT).

        a. Cone-beam computed tomography (CBCT) systems are a variation of traditional computed tomography (CT) systems. The CBCT systems used by dental professionals rotate around the patient, capturing data using a cone-shaped x-ray beam. These data are used to reconstruct a three-dimensional (3D) image of the following regions of the patient's anatomy: dental (teeth); oral and maxillofacial region (mouth, jaw, and neck); and ears, nose, and throat (ENT).

2. The dental assistant should be able to demonstrate basic knowledge of digital radiography and other modern imaging techniques.

    a. advantages of digital radiography

        i. immediate feedback on exposure
        ii. patients receive a considerably smaller amount of radiation exposure
        iii. eliminates the need for developer and fixer in the office
        iv. images can be readily emailed to referral offices or insurance companies

    b. disadvantages of digital radiography

        i. sensors are rigid and take practice to place without discomfort to patient
        ii. sensors are expensive and require delicate handling
        iii. assistant must learn radiography software in order to produce diagnostic-quality radiographs
        iv. If the computer is not working for whatever reason, you cannot take radiographs.

    c. The dental assistant should understand handling errors and how to avoid them. Know how to avoid mistakes and, when mistakes are made, how to quickly correct them for a diagnostic quality radiographs.

    d. General considerations for digital radiography sensors/imaging plates

        i. Digital radiography sensors/imaging plates come into contact with mucous membranes and are considered semicritical devices. Ideally, they should be cleaned and heat sterilized or high-level disinfected between patients.
        ii. Currently, the sensors/plates cannot withstand heat sterilization or complete immersion in a high-level disinfectant. Therefore, these devices should, at a minimum, be covered with an FDA-cleared barrier and then, according to the Centers for Disease Control and Prevention, the sensor/plates should be cleaned and disinfected with an EPA-registered intermediate-level disinfectant after the barrier has been removed and discarded.

    e. Digital radiographic positioning devices

        i. Most, if not all, positioning devices such as Snap-A-Rays or Rinn holders are heat tolerant.

            a. Before reuse on a patient, clean, package, and heat sterilize.

            b. Disposable positioning devices are used once and discarded.

        ii. general considerations for managing computers and related equipment in the dental operatory

            a. Avoiding contamination is important because many items cannot be properly cleaned and disinfected or sterilized. Good hand hygiene is important. Before touching any office equipment, ensure your hands are clean, and if wearing gloves, select a powder-free brand.

            b. The basic principles of cleaning and disinfection used routinely in the dental operatory also apply to computer equipment. Computer equipment is considered a clinical contact surface. Therefore, if the potential for contamination exists, use plastic protective surface barriers to prevent contamination.

            c. To minimize the potential for patient cross-contamination of the computer keyboard and mouse, adequately cover all surfaces with plastic barriers that will be contacted with gloved or contaminated hands or that may be contaminated by spatter/spray.

d. Barrier examples for the computer keyboard include single-use plastic disposable covers such as a headrest cover or plastic wrap or preformed plastic keyboard covers that can be removed and cleaned.

e. Barrier examples for the computer mouse include single-use plastic self-adhesive sheets or overgloves.

3. The dental assistant should demonstrate knowledge of conventional film processing.

   a. Describe functions of processing solutions and procedures for maintaining integrity of processing solutions.

      i. **Fixer** is the solution used in film processing that stops the action of the developer and makes the radiographic image permanently visible. It should be replenished each day and replaced each week. Most fixer comes premixed in a container. Some products are sold in powder form, and the user is responsible for proper mixing with water following the manufacturer's instructions. Used fixer must be stored in an EPA-approved container and picked up by a licensed hauler. Fixer contains silver halide crystals, which are removed from the film, and is detrimental to the environment if placed down the drain. Never dispose of fixer in any other manner.

      ii. **Developer** is the solution used in film processing that makes the radiographic image latent. It should be replenished daily and replaced weekly. Most developer comes premixed in a container. Some products are sold in powder form, and the user is responsible for proper mixing with water following the manufacturer's instructions. Developer may be disposed of down the drain and is not harmful to the environment.

      iii. Never add more water to correctly mixed or premixed developer or fixer in an attempt to "top off" containers. This decreases the integrity of the chemicals and can render them unusable. Only "top off" solution containers with appropriately mixed or premixed solutions or **replenisher**.

   b. The assistant should be aware of how to process intra- and extraoral radiographs by use of manual and automatic techniques.

   c. Optimum conditions for processing radiographs such as proper processing temperatures and chemical mixtures if using dip tanks or processors, exposure times, and kVp settings must be observed.

      i. The x-ray tube contains either a filament or cathode emitter that expels accelerated electrons and leads them to a metal anode, where current is now flowing. The electrons that have been emitted toward the anode make up an electron beam. The beam hits a focal point in the anode, where a small percentage is converted into x-ray photons. The photons are discharged in all directions, and once the control unit is put to use, the adjusted currents and voltage result in a beam of x-rays that is projected onto a visible substance. An x-ray machine essentially acts as a camera, but without the visible light. Instead, it uses the x-rays that were produced to expose the film. X-rays use electromagnetic waves that can break through several layers due to the energy held inside them. If the body is being x-rayed, the skin tissue will not absorb the waves coming from the x-ray, but the dense parts of the body will, which is why bones, tendons, and ligaments are able to be examined.

C. Evaluate

1. The dental assistant should be able to evaluate radiographs for diagnostic value.

   a. Diagnostically acceptable radiographic images include properly placed film to capture the area of interest with no cone cuts, proper exposure times, images that are clear, and images that do not have elongations or foreshortened exposures or overlapping.

   b. Identify and describe common errors related to acquiring radiographic images.

      i. Film distortion is best described as any film placement that results in a less-than-ideal relationship between the film and x-ray position indicating device that results in an image that is not diagnostically readable (Figure 2-7).

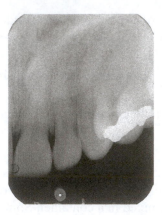

Figure 2-7 A curved film distorts radiograph images.

ii. elongation – This refers to a distortion of the image in which the tooth structures appear longer than the anatomical size. This is usually caused by insufficient vertical angulation of the central beam (Figure 2-8).

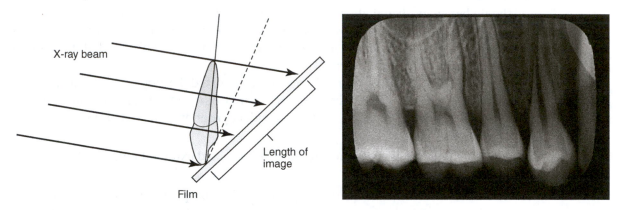

Figure 2-8 Elongation on a radiograph

iii. foreshortening – This refers to a distortion of the image in which the tooth structures appear shorter than their actual anatomical size. This is most often caused by excessive vertical angulation of the central beam (Figure 2-9).

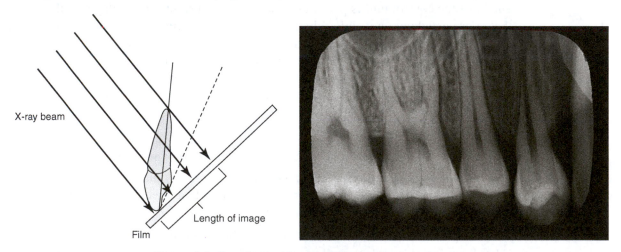

Figure 2-9 Foreshortening on a radiograph

iv. horizontal overlapping – occurs when horizontal angulation causes the primary beam to create an overlapping of the teeth and the interproximal areas are not seen (Figure 2-10)

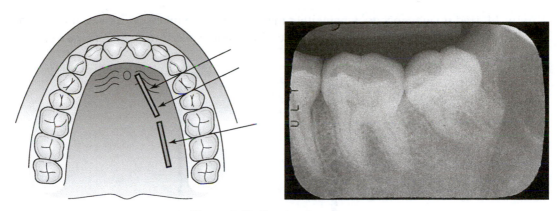

Figure 2-10 Overlapping

v. cone cutting – This occurs when the primary beam is not centered on the film and produces a blank or clear area in that part of the radiograph (Figure 2-11).

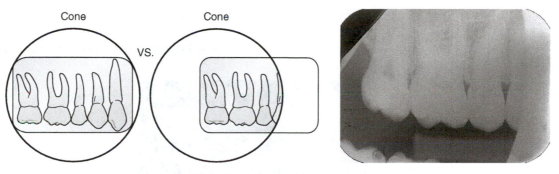

Figure 2-11 Cone cutting

vi. blank or clear film – film was not exposed to enough radiation (Figure 2-12)

Figure 2-12 Clear film

vii. double exposure – occurs when the film is exposed twice (Figure 2-13)

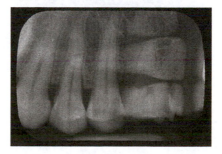

Figure 2-13 Double exposure

viii. blurred image – occurs when either the subject or the tubehead moves during exposure
xi. underexposed film – occurs when the film is not exposed to radiation and appears too light (Figure 2-14)

Figure 2-14 Underexposed film

x. overexposed film – occurs when the film is exposed to too much radiation and appears too dark (Figure 2-15)

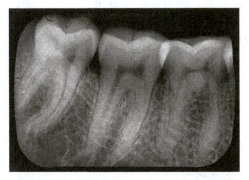

Figure 2-15 Overexposed film

xi. film artifact – occurs when there is a bend in the film or there is an item that appears on the film that is not part of the human anatomy and is reflected on the radiograph as part of the image (Figure 2-16)

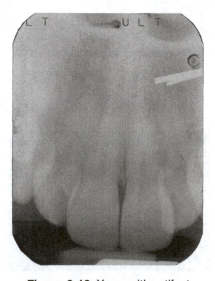

Figure 2-16 X-ray with artifact

xii. backward film (herringbone effect) – occurs when the film is placed backward in the patient's mouth (Figure 2-17)

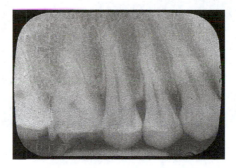

Figure 2-17 Herringbone effect

c. Identify and describe common errors related to processing radiographic images.

i. light image – Film may not have been processed long enough in the developer or was not exposed long enough to radiation (Figure 2-18).

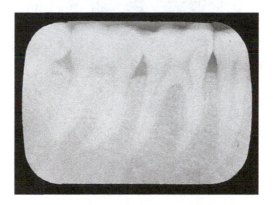

Figure 2-18 Light image on radiograph

ii. dark image – Film may have been overprocessed or overexposed (Figure 2-19).

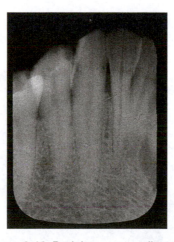

Figure 2-19 Dark image on radiograph

iii. fogged film – *Fogged films* have a gray appearance, image detail is lost, and contrast is lessened (Figure 2-20).

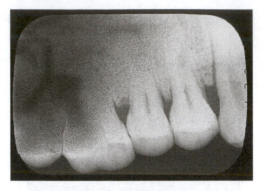

Figure 2-20 Fogged film

iv. partial image – This will occur when dental appliances, body piercings, or jewelry exposure will appear as radiopaque artifacts superimposed over the dental image (Figure 2-21).

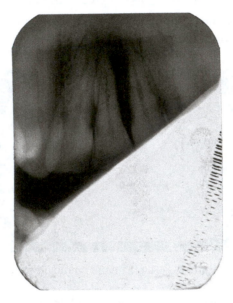

Figure 2-21 Partial image due to low levels of processing solution

v. spotted film – This occurs when film is processed using chemicals and developer or fixer is splashed on the film during processing (Figure 2-22 and 2-23).

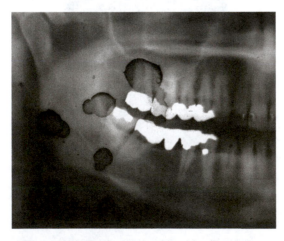

Figure 2-22 Radiograph with white (fixer) spots

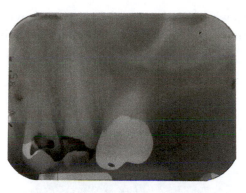

Figure 2-23 Radiograph with dark (developer) spots

     vi. air bubbles on film – This can occur during chemical processing when the film is placed in the rinse and then developer without agitating the film. The water bubbles remain on the film when developer is introduced (Figure 2-24).

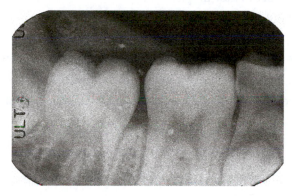

Figure 2-24 Air bubbles on radiograph

     vii. reticulation – occurs when the film is subjected to a sudden temperature change between the developer and water during processing, which results in a cracked appearance
    viii. black film – film was exposed to visible light

 d. Identify and describe common errors related to improper handling of radiographic images
      i. torn or scratched film
     ii. white or black lines
    iii. static electricity artifacts
    iv. fingerprints (Figure 2-25)

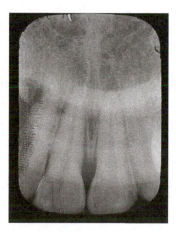

Figure 2-25 Fingerprint on radiograph

v. film bending – occurs when film is bent while either removing from film packet, moving through the processor, or during film placement in the mouth. Black lines will be present where film was bent (Figure 2-26).

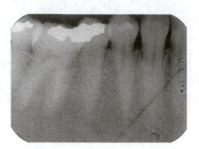

Figure 2-26 Bent film artifact

    vi. film placement errors – General placement errors occur when film is placed in incorrect positions and misses the subject matter in question.

e. The dental assistant should be able to identify and correct common errors when exposing panoramic radiographs to include patient positioning errors.

    i. Overall grayness or blackness along one edge or corner of film (fog)

        a. cause: damaged cassette (light leak) or film exposed to light

        b. correction: tape edges of soft cassette or replace damaged hard cassette

    ii. Little or no image is visible on film

        a. cause: screens reversed

        b. correction: replace screens properly

    iii. Black marks, round clusters or lightning-bolt image

        a. cause: static electricity

        b. correction: remove film slowly from the film cassette prior to processing

    iv. Multiple images

        a. cause: double exposure

        b. correction: remove film cassette after each exposure and store exposed and unexposed film separately

    v. White streaks on image

        a. cause: scratched or damaged screens

        b. correction: handle screens and clean carefully with a soft cloth or replace with new screens if too damaged

    vi. Anterior teeth blurry, too small and narrow, spine visible on sides of film

        a. cause: patient is biting too far forward on bite rod

        b. correction: make certain anterior teeth are located in the grooves on rod

    vii. Anterior teeth blurry and wide, ghosting of mandible and spine, condyles close to edge of film

        a. cause: patient is biting too far back on rod or not at all

        b. correction: make certain anterior teeth are located in grooves on rod

    viii. White tapered opacity in middle of image

        a. cause: ghost of spinal column due to slumping

        b. correction: have patient take a step forward and straighten spine and neck

       ix. Large, dark shadow over maxillary teeth between palate and dorsum of tongue

          a. cause: patient tongue not in roof of mouth

          b. correction: ask patient to swallow and place tongue on roof of mouth

       x. White vertical line on film running from top to bottom edge of film

          a. cause: exposure stopped briefly, most likely due to letting go of the exposure button

          b. correction: Most machines will return to start position if this occurs. Re-expose panoramic radiograph.

2. Mounting and Labeling Radiographs

   a. Describe how to mount radiographs using facial (buccal and labial) view.

      i. The dental assistant should be able to identify anatomical landmarks that aid in the correct mounting of radiographs. Anatomical landmarks include sinuses and the V-shaped structure that is the nasal septum, alveolar crest, roots, and general shape of the tooth.

         a. Landmarks of the maxilla include the nasal septum, anterior nasal spine, septum, zygomatic process of the maxilla, maxillary tuberosity, hamular process, maxillary sinus, and incisive foramen.

         b. Landmarks of the mandibular area include the lingual foramen, mental foramen, mental fossa, mandibular nerve canal, genial tubercle, and mylohyoid ridge.

         c. Landmarks of the face may include the tragus of the ear, the ala of the nose, or the orbital sockets of the eye.

     ii. The dental assistant should be able to mount specific tooth views to specified tooth mount windows.

         a. Tooth views include the buccal and lingual views. Buccal view is viewed as if you are facing the patient and looking at them; your right is their left and vice versa. The lingual view would be viewed as if you are sitting on the patient's tongue looking outward, so your left side would be the patient's left side.

         b. The assistant should be able to use a full-mouth as well as a bitewing mount to place radiographs in proper sequence for viewing. Anterior radiographs are located in the center open areas, while the posterior radiographs are mounted on the periphery, with the most posterior views located on the outside. This mimics the patient's dentition and makes diagnosis and interpretation easier.

         c. Roots and crowns of the maxillary anterior teeth are larger than those of the mandibular teeth, while maxillary molars generally have three roots and the mandibular molars only have two roots. Most roots will curve toward the distal, and the body of the mandible has a distinct upward curve toward the ramus in the molar area.

         d. Using identification dots is crucial in the proper mounting of radiographs. Depending on your office and where your dentist graduated, all dots will be either convex or concave when mounting. Radiographs taken digitally do not require this.

         e. Sometimes a coin envelope is used for duplicates or single radiographs. The coin envelope should include the patient's name, date radiograph was taken, and dentist's name. It is also helpful if the tooth or teeth numbers are listed on the envelope as well.

    iii. The dental assistant should be able to demonstrate appropriate techniques for optimum viewing.

         a. Using a view box is the best way to examine radiographs. If a view box is not available, holding the radiographs up to the operatory light can give you an adequate view of the radiograph. When using digital radiographs, the assistant should be able to manipulate the computer's contrast button to bring the radiograph into adequate viewing.

         b. A magnifying glass is also helpful when trying to focus on details in the radiograph.

         c. Try to diminish as much excess light as possible when viewing radiographs.

b. Identification of anatomical structures, dental materials, and patient information observed on radiographs

   i. The dental assistant should be able to differentiate between radiopaque and radiolucent areas of the radiographs. Radiolucent are any darker areas on the radiograph, while lighter or clear areas are referred to as radiopaque.

      a. Radiopaque items that can appear on a radiograph include bone, amalgam, enamel, gutta percha, pins, crowns with metal in them, and any hard-tissue anomalies.

      b. Radiolucent items that can appear on a radiograph include sinus areas, abscesses, and any soft-tissue anomalies.

D. Patient Management

   1. The dental assistant should be able to select patient-management techniques before, during, and after radiographic exposure such as addressing patient concerns about radiation, exposing radiographs, and patient refusal of radiographs.

      a. Often patients can become concerned about the amount of exposure they are receiving. It is important to convey to the patient that you are using high-speed film and a lead apron and exposing as few radiographs as possible. If you use digital radiographs in the practice you work in, explain to the patient the benefits of digital radiographs and their lower emission of radiation.

      b. Fear toward radiation and dental radiographs can lead to patient refusal of radiographs. It is always important to reassure the patient that you will be taking only the radiographs needed and that the dentist must have them to accurately diagnose and treat their dental condition. Never ask a patient to sign a refusal for radiographs, because that is nothing more than informed neglect. It will not help you in a court of law. Sometimes it is better to dismiss the patient from the practice and record accurate notes of the patient's refusal.

      c. On occasion, you may see a patient who is mentally or physically disabled. If a patient is hard of hearing, then writing your request or making gestures may be an option. If a patient is blind, they may need you to explain in more detail what you plan to do and how they can help you. When a patient physically cannot get into the chair, it is possible to expose radiographs while they are seated in their wheelchair. Helping the patient get into the dental chair may be an option if the patient is willing to let you do this.

   2. The patient who gags is stimulated by both psychological as well as tactile stimuli. The thought of having something placed in the back of the throat alone can cause the activation of the gag reflex. Giving the patient a task to perform such as holding the film holder or asking them to breathe deeply during film placement will put the patient's mind somewhere else. Also, anesthetic spray can reduce the sensitivity of the gag reflex.

   3. Patients with mental disabilities require more patience. Oftentimes, mentally disabled patients will have a caregiver with them who can help you by giving the patient directions or by helping the patient perform simple tasks.

Important Objectives to Know

- Be able to describe the functions of processing solutions.
- Understand the process of exposing intra- and extraoral radiographs by use of manual and automatic techniques.
- Be able to mount radiographs using the buccal view.
- Identify anatomical landmarks that aid correct mounting.
- Be able to match specific tooth views to specified tooth mount windows.
- Demonstrate appropriate techniques for optimum viewing.
- Identify anatomical structures, dental materials, and patient information.
- Be able to differentiate between radiopaque and radiolucent.
- Identify which structures in the radiograph would appear radiolucent or radiopaque.

Study Checklist

1. Review text chapter on radiology.
2. Review all terminology related to radiographic exposure.
3. Review text regarding special-needs patients and radiation exposure.
4. Review oral anatomy and dentition.

Section I:
Expose and Evaluate – Review Questions

Use the Answer Sheet found in Appendix A.

1. Which term describes the white areas on the processed radiograph?
   a. density
   b. penumbra
   c. radiolucent
   d. radiopaque

2. Subject contrast is affected by
   a. processing procedures.
   b. type of film.
   c. scatter radiation.
   d. crystal size.

3. Which term best describes the amount of light transmitted through a film?
   a. definition
   b. contrast
   c. density
   d. penetration

4. Which factor has the greatest effect on film sharpness?
   a. movement
   b. filtration
   c. kilovoltage
   d. amperage

5. Distortion is caused when
   a. object and film are parallel.
   b. object and film are not parallel.
   c. using a short object-film distance.
   d. using a long target-film distance.

6. The dental radiograph will appear lighter if one increases the
   a. mA.
   b. kVp.
   c. exposure time.
   d. target-film distance.

7. Selection of proper kVp is influenced most by which two of the following?
   a. size of film
   b. size of patient and density of tissues
   c. developing temperature
   d. distance of tubehead to patient

8. The film most likely to initiate the gag reflex is
   a. maxillary premolar.
   b. maxillary molar.
   c. mandibular premolar.
   d. mandibular molar.

9. All of the following are advantages to using digital radiographs except which one?
   a. less radiation exposure to the patient
   b. film sensor is larger
   c. no need for developer and fixer in the office
   d. you are able to see the image immediately

10. Your dentist asks you to expose a periapical radiograph showing the mesial of #3, and after exposing the radiograph, you observe overlapping. The most likely cause is
    a. too much vertical angulation.
    b. radiograph not in the path of the primary beam.
    c. too much horizontal angulation.
    d. too little exposure in interproximal areas.

11. Film placement for a patient with palatal torus is
    a. between the torus and the tongue.
    b. on the top of the torus.
    c. on the near side of the torus, close to the teeth.
    d. on the far side of the torus, away from the teeth.

12. Film placement for a patient with a mandibular torus is:
    a. on top of the torus.
    b. on top of the tongue.
    c. between the torus and the tongue.
    d. none of the above.

13. Why is patient education in radiography necessary?
    a. to increase the demand for radiographic services
    b. because it is legally required
    c. to assure the patient that all radiographers are licensed
    d. because patients must be reassured that dental radiation procedures are safe

14. Which of these is not a method of patient education in radiography?
    a. information given orally at chairside
    b. follow-up letters from the dentist
    c. visual presentation of enlarged radiographs
    d. pamphlets on radiation protection

15. What does a diamond or herringbone pattern on the processed radiograph indicate?
    a. expired film
    b. underexposed film
    c. reversed film
    d. overdeveloped film

16. Which of these conditions is caused by insufficient vertical angulation?
    a. elongation
    b. overlapping

c. foreshortening

d. cone cutting

17. Which of these conditions results from a failure to direct the central ray toward the middle of the film packet?

a. cone cut

b. overlapping

c. elongation

d. foreshadowing

18. Which of these indicates that the radiograph was overexposed?

a. light image

b. reticulation

c. dark image

d. thin black lines

19. Which of these indicates that the film was not properly washed?

a. light image

b. fogging

c. brownish-yellow

d. white spots

20. Which of these is not a cause of fogging of the radiograph?

a. exposure to scatter radiation

b. exposure to white light

c. overexposure

d. chemical fog

21. What is the probable cause of reticulation?

a. overexposure

b. underexposure

c. differences in processing solution temperatures

d. cracks in the safelight

22. How will static electricity appear radiographically?

a. as black lines

b. as a brownish-yellow stain

c. as white lines

d. as fog

23. Which of these items appears radiolucent?

a. enamel

b. dental pulp

c. bone

d. dentin

24. Why would a film appear blank?

a. It was not exposed to fixer.

b. It was not exposed to radiation.

c. It was not exposed to developer.

d. It was exposed to heat.

25. Which type of crystals are embedded in the emulsion on the film that affects the speed or sensitivity of the film?

a. halide

b. bromide

c. fluorine

d. radioresistant

26. If a patient refuses radiographs, the best course of action would be for the office to what?

a. Request that the patient sign a waiver stating they do not want radiographs.

b. Take the radiographs anyway.

c. Explain to the patient that the dentist cannot perform an accurate exam without them.

d. After counseling the patient and still they refuse, excuse the patient from practice.

27. The lead foil found within the film packet is designed to accomplish what function?

a. It is used to absorb some of the radiation that passes through the film and helps prevent scatter of radiation to the surrounding tissue.

b. It is used to absorb heat generated by the gamma rays generated within the tubehead.

c. It is designed to deflect hard rays that are not useful in exposing radiographs.

d. It is provided to increase flexibility of the film packet.

28. According to ANSI, which film would be considered the fastest speed?

a. A

b. B

c. D

d. E

29. Using a long cone will produce exposures that

a. are sharper than film exposed using a short cone.

b. are less sharp than film exposed using a short cone.

c. are darker than an exposure using a short cone.

d. are more diagnostically accurate than an exposure using a short cone.

30. When taking digital radiographs, the BEST way to minimize the potential for patient cross-contamination of the computer keyboard and mouse is to

a. wipe down with an EPA-registered disinfectant after each use.

b. adequately cover all surfaces with plastic barriers that will be contacted with gloved or contaminated hands.

c. have a coworker help you by using the keyboard and mouse with clean hands.

d. use an overglove when touching the mouse or keyboard.

31. The best infection control for digital sensors is to

a. place in the autoclave.

b. place in the dry heat sterilizer.

c. place in the chemclave.

d. wipe clean with a hospital-grade disinfectant with no more than 80% alcohol.

32. Which of these terms describes the ability to read a radiograph?

a. case presentation

b. prognosis

c. dissertation

d. interpretation

33. Which of these is a facial landmark?
    a. coronoid process
    b. glenoid fossa
    c. tragus
    d. mylohyoid ridge

34. Which of these is not a mandibular landmark?
    a. incisive foramen
    b. lingual foramen
    c. coronoid process
    d. mental foramen

35. Which of these structures appears radiolucent?
    a. enamel
    b. dental pulp
    c. dentin
    d. alveolar process

36. Which of these structures appears radiopaque?
    a. maxillary sinus
    b. nasal fossa
    c. maxillary tuberosity
    d. mental foramen

37. Which of these appears most radiopaque?
    a. trabecular bone
    b. cementum
    c. dentin
    d. enamel

38. A bony projection that extends downward and slightly posterior in many maxillary molar radiographs is the
    a. mastoid process.
    b. styloid process.
    c. condylar process.
    d. hamular process.

39. In a radiograph of the maxillary molars, the following structure may obscure the roots of the teeth.
    a. zygomatic process of the maxilla
    b. maxillary tuberosity
    c. mastoid process
    d. mylohyoid ridge

40. Most dental schools now teach that for viewing, radiographs should be mounted as though
    a. you are seated on the tongue looking out.
    b. you are facing the patient.
    c. you are viewing the patient from behind.
    d. you are viewing the patient from the side.

41. Which of these helps determine whether the radiograph is of the patient's right or left side?
    a. lamina dura
    b. film emulsion
    c. location of the septum
    d. identification dot

42. When new radiographs are taken, the previous radiographs are
    a. sent to the patient.
    b. discarded.

c. placed in a coin envelope, labeled, and kept in the patient file.
    d. stored in another location other than the dental office.

43. Whom do the original radiographs belong to?
    a. the patient
    b. the office
    c. the insurance company since they paid for them
    d. the dental board

44. A patient is entitled to a copy of their radiographs
    a. free of charge.
    b. only after they have a zero account balance.
    c. upon request.
    d. never; they are the property of the dental office not the patient.

45. Which item appears radiolucent on a radiograph?
    a. enamel
    b. periapical abscess
    c. trabecular bone
    d. amalgam filling

46. Mounting radiographs while the dot is convex tells the evaluator that
    a. they are viewing the patient's dentition as though they are sitting on the patient's tongue looking out.
    b. they are viewing the patient's dentition as though they are facing the patient.
    c. the radiographs are one dimensional.
    d. the dot makes no difference whether it convex or concave.

47. A radiolucent mandibular landmark that can be seen around the first and second bicuspid is
    a. the mandibular foramen.
    b. genial tubercles.
    c. mandibular canal.
    d. mandibular tori.

48. The pulp of the tooth on a radiograph appears
    a. radiopaque.
    b. radiolucent.
    c. grainy.
    d. reticulated.

49. The doughnut-shaped bony crests on the lingual surface of the mandible are referred to as
    a. tori.
    b. genial tubercles.
    c. mental ridge.
    d. retromolar area.

50. The V-shaped projection from the floor of the nasal fossa in the midline is referred to as the
    a. nasal septum.
    b. maxillary tuberosity.
    c. anterior nasal spine.
    d. zygomatic arch.

51. Legal reasons radiographs should be taken may include
    a. accurate diagnostic purposes.
    b. insurance records.

c. compare to past restorative work.
d. all of the above.

52. At the minimum, by law, the following items should appear on a radiograph mount:
    a. patient's name, date, and dentist's name.
    b. patient's name, birthday, and tooth in question.
    c. patient's name, address, and chart number.
    d. patient's name, tooth pictured in radiograph, and date.

53. Where should materials designed to absorb primary and secondary radiation be installed?
    a. walls, floor, and ceiling
    b. walls, floor, and doors
    c. floor, walls, and door
    d. walls, door, and ceiling

54. Which of the following film requires the least exposure time?
    a. D-speed
    b. E-speed
    c. F-speed
    d. Ultraspeed

55. If a patient cannot hold the film or sensor in their mouth during exposure, the best way to stabilize the sensor or the film would be to do the following:
    a. Hold the sensor or film for the patient.
    b. Have a family member hold the sensor or film.
    c. Have the patient hold the sensor or film.
    d. Use a hemostat.

56. Film that has a herringbone effect after processing has what type of exposure error?
    a. Film was processed at too high a temperature.
    b. Film was exposed facing backward in the patient's mouth.
    c. Film was bent during developing.
    d. Film was exposed to heat before use.

57. When reading radiographs, density can be defined as
    a. sharpness.
    b. clarity.
    c. the amount of light transmitted through a film.
    d. blurriness.

58. In radiographic exposure, the differences between light and dark shades is known as
    a. cumulative.
    b. isolated.
    c. temporary.
    d. transient.

59. Film sizes range between 0 and 4. Which number corresponds to the occlusal film?
    a. 0
    b. 1
    c. 2
    d. 4

60. A film that appears too dark is a result of which action taking place?
    a. underexposed
    b. overlapped

c. not exposed to radiation
d. overexposure

61. When exposing radiographs, blurred images are a result of
    a. tubehead or patient movement during exposure.
    b. processing at high temperatures.
    c. double exposure.
    d. too much vertical angulation.

62. During radiographic exposure, too much vertical angulation can result in
    a. overlapping.
    b. elongation.
    c. cone cutting.
    d. foreshortening.

63. When mounting radiographic films, the ADA recommends that you mount the dots out. Which type of view of the patient would this indicate?
    a. The patient is facing the operator.
    b. The patient has their back to the operator.
    c. The dot does not make a difference.
    d. The patient is parallel to the operator.

64. A panoramic radiograph takes a recording of which areas?
    a. just the interproximal areas of the teeth
    b. the entire maxilla and mandible in one picture
    c. the occlusal and incisal portion of the teeth
    d. only the maxilla and nasal areas

65. The best film to use to detect interproximal carious lesions is referred to as what?
    a. periapical
    b. panoramic
    c. occlusal
    d. bitewing

66. If a patient presents with a possible abscess at the apex of the tooth, the best diagnostic radiograph to take for the operator to read would be which of the following radiographs?
    a. bitewing
    b. occlusal
    c. periapical
    d. panoramic

67. Films that are processed that show the teeth elongated can be remedied by moving the position indicating device (PID) in which direction?
    a. horizontally
    b. vertically
    c. to the left of the patient
    d. to the right of the patient

68. Film artifacts are best described as what?
    a. fingerprints or smudge marks
    b. air bubbles
    c. torn or scratched film
    d. any of the above

69. When referring to radiopacity on a radiographic film, you are talking about what?
    a. the darkness of the radiograph
    b. the density of the radiograph

c. the sharpness of the radiograph

d. the lightness or clear areas of the image on the radiograph

70. Which of the following are indications for radiographs?
    a. to detect bone loss
    b. to detect carious lesions
    c. for evaluation prior to oral surgery
    d. Any of the above can be indications to take a radiograph.

71. The _____ the film or sensor stays in the patient's mouth prior to exposure, the less likely the patient is to gag.
    a. more
    b. less
    c. both
    d. neither

72. On a periapical radiograph, what is the small circular radiolucency near the roots of the mandibular premolars?
    a. lingual foramen
    b. mental foramen
    c. mandibular foramen
    d. incisive foramen

73. After processing a film, it comes out clear. This could be from which error?
    a. overexposure
    b. improper chemical temperatures
    c. film was not exposed to radiation
    d. film was in the fixer too long

74. A cone cut is a result of which exposure error?
    a. having incorrect horizontal angulation
    b. not being aimed at the collimator
    c. having increased vertical angulation
    d. primary beam not being aimed at the center of the film

75. When positioning a patient for a panoramic radiograph, the following should be removed:
    a. earrings.
    b. partials or dentures.
    c. eyewear such as glasses.
    d. any or all of the above.

76. An amalgam restoration will appear as what type of image?
    a. radiolucent
    b. radiopaque
    c. encapsulated
    d. herringbone pattern

77. Fogged dental radiography film can be caused by what?
    a. exposure to heat
    b. exposure to light
    c. outdated film
    d. any of the above

78. Radiographic technique for exposing the edentulous survey requires which of the following?
    a. using cotton rolls and Styrofoam blocks
    b. substituting the alveolar ridge for the long axis of the missing tooth
    c. using a lower exposure time
    d. Any of the above can be used when exposing radiographs on the edentulous patient.

79. The number of exposures that comprise an adult full-mouth series is considered to be how many exposures?
    a. 18–20 exposures
    b. 10–15 exposures
    c. 20–25 exposures
    d. 14–16 exposures

80. When processing, a film that appears too dark is a result of what error occurring?
    a. underexposure
    b. overexposure
    c. cold fixer
    d. rinse not agitated

81. The advantage of increasing the target-film distance for patient protection is that it serves to accomplish what action?
    a. increases scatter radiation
    b. reduces film speed
    c. decreases radiation intensity
    d. It doesn't accomplish any of the above.

82. The function of an intensifying screen is designed to accomplish which task?
    a. It is the hard container that holds the film.
    b. It is used to intensify the action of the x-ray.
    c. It is held by the patient during exposure.
    d. It is the two screens that appear on each side of the film and is used to intensify the action of the x-rays to decrease exposure to the patient.

83. Extraoral films are utilized for which purpose?
    a. viewing the skull
    b. detecting fractures
    c. detecting anomalies
    d. An extraoral film can be used for any of the above reasons.

84. After processing a film, you notice a lightning bolt effect on the film. This is caused by what?
    a. static electricity
    b. milliamperage (mA) is set too high
    c. overexposure
    d. improper fixer temperature

85. The dark areas of the radiograph are referred to as what?
    a. contrasting
    b. radiolucent
    c. radiopaque
    d. dense

86. What is the best way to place film or a sensor on a patient who has mandibular tori?
    a. on top of the torus
    b. on top of the tongue
    c. between the torus and the tongue
    d. none of the above

87. A latent image can best be described as what?
    a. an unseen image that is on the film from exposure time until the image is processed
    b. an image that appears after the film has been processed
    c. an image that is blurry
    d. an image stored and used at a later date

88. Detail of radiographs can be best described as what?
    a. varying degrees of shades of gray present in the image
    b. the degree of darkness in the image
    c. the degree of radiopacity
    d. the degree of sharpness or clarity of image

89. A cephalometric radiograph is primarily used for which specialty?
    a. endodontics
    b. periodontics
    c. oral surgery
    d. orthodontics

90. Which factor has the greatest effect on film sharpness?
    a. movement
    b. filtration
    c. kilovoltage
    d. amperage

91. When does distortion of an x-ray occur?
    a. object and film are parallel
    b. object and film are not parallel
    c. using a short object-film distance
    d. using a long target-film distance

92. Which is most likely to produce a radiograph with long-scale contrast?
    a. when kVp is increased
    b. when kVp is decreased
    c. when mAs are increased
    d. when mAs are decreased

93. The dental radiograph will appear lighter if the operator increases which setting?
    a. mA
    b. kVp
    c. exposure time
    d. film distance

94. What is the purpose of the lead foil in the x-ray film packet?
    a. moisture protection
    b. absorb the backscatter radiation
    c. to give rigidity to the packet
    d. protection against fluorescence

95. Which film is placed outside the mouth during an x-ray exposure?
    a. occlusal film
    b. periapical film
    c. intraoral film
    d. extraoral film

96. Which of these films uses the shortest exposure time?
    a. nonscreen film
    b. screen film
    c. panoramic film
    d. duplicating film

97. Which type of film is used to copy a radiograph?
    a. duplicating film
    b. screen film
    c. nonscreen film
    d. x-ray film

98. Which term best describes the process by which the latent image becomes visible?
    a. reticulation
    b. reduction
    c. sensitivity
    d. preservation

99. Which term describes a fully processed radiograph that shows a network of cracks on its surface?
    a. fogged
    b. reticulated
    c. restrained
    d. proliferated

100. A panoramic radiograph is of little value when diagnosing which condition?
    a. an impacted molar
    b. recurrent caries
    c. a cyst
    d. sinus deformities

101. Replenisher is added to the developing solution to accomplish what?
    a. compensate for oxidation
    b. compensate for loss of volume
    c. compensate for loss of solution strength
    d. Addition of developing solution can be added to accomplish any of the above.

102. The processing tank should be cleaned at what intervals?
    a. every day
    b. once a week
    c. every two weeks
    d. whenever the solutions are changed

103. Which of the following appears more radiopaque?
    a. bone
    b. cementum
    c. pulp
    d. amalgam

104. Which of these helps determine whether a radiograph exposure is on the patient's left or right?
    a. lamina dura
    b. film emulsion
    c. location of the septum
    d. identification dot

105. Caries or decay in its first stages of existence is called what?
    a. senile caries
    b. class I caries
    c. incipient caries
    d. primary decay

106. Caries that occurs under a restoration or around the margin of an existing crown is referred to as which type of decay?
    a. recurrent caries
    b. dentinal caries
    c. root caries
    d. buccal caries

107. Which of these materials appears most radiolucent on a radiograph?
    a. amalgam
    b. dental porcelain
    c. silicate
    d. acrylic resin

108. A Rinn film holder is helpful in avoiding which radiographic exposure mistake?
    a. conecutting
    b. overlapping
    c. elongation
    d. Any of the above can be avoided using a Rinn holder.

109. In radiography, a partial shadow or fuzzy outline around the image is referred to as what?
    a. penumbra
    b. overlapping
    c. mutations
    d. light fog

Section I:
Expose and Evaluate – Answers and Rationales

1. Which term describes the white areas on the processed radiograph?

   d. radiopaque – is the term that is used to describe the "white" or opaque areas on a radiographic film. The denser material, such as bone, will appear radiopaque.

2. Subject contrast is affected by

   c. scatter radiation – Each patient or "subject" exhibits different rates of absorption with the different tissues being exposed. Patients have contrast because each person has tissues that vary in thickness and size. Scatter radiation interacts with these tissues, which can influence "subject" contrast, NOT film contrast. That is different.

3. Which term best describes the amount of light transmitted through a film?

   d. penetration – This is the ability of light to transmit through the film.

4. Which factor has the greatest effect on film sharpness?

   a. movement – The movement of a patient or the tubehead during exposure greatly affects the sharpness of a processed film.

5. Distortion is caused when

   b. object and film are not parallel – When the film and the object are NOT parallel, distortion may occur such as elongation or foreshortening.

6. The dental radiograph will appear lighter if one increases the

   d. target-film distance – The image on a processed radiograph will appear lighter if there is more distance between the target or patient and the film.

7. Selection of proper kVp is influenced most by which two of the following?

   b. size of patient and density of tissues – kVp determines the quality of the radiograph, so patient tissues and size affect the density. The more the kVp is increased, the shorter the wavelength and the higher the energy and penetrating power of the x-rays produced.

8. The film most likely to initiate the gag reflex is

   b. maxillary molar

9. All of the following are advantages to using digital radiographs except which one?

   b. film sensor is larger

10. Your dentist asks you to expose a periapical radiograph showing the mesial of #3, and after exposing the radiograph, you observe overlapping. The most likely cause is

    c. too much horizontal angulation.

11. Film placement for a patient with palatal torus should be

    d. on the far side of the torus, away from the teeth – This provides maximum comfort for the patient.

12. Film placement for a patient with a mandibular torus is

    c. between the torus and the tongue – The tongue acts as a cushion for the patient to cushion the rigidity of the film against the tori.

13. Why is patient education in radiography necessary?

    d. because patients must be reassured that dental radiation procedures are safe – Patients must be reassured that taking radiographs is both a necessity for complete diagnosis and they are safe when proper shielding and safety devices are in place.

14. Which of these is not a method of patient education in radiography?

    b. follow-up letters from the dentist – A follow-up letter only reveals the findings of an already exposed radiograph, not the safety advantages of taking radiographs.

15. What does a diamond or herringbone pattern on the processed radiograph indicate?

    c. reversed film – When a film is reversed in the mouth, the lead shield, which has a herringbone pattern, is visible. The smooth, flat portion of the radiograph must face the outside of the mouth to prevent this herringbone effect from occurring.

16. Which of these conditions is caused by insufficient vertical angulation?

    a. elongation

17. Which of these conditions results from a failure to direct the central ray toward the middle of the film packet?

    a. cone cut – A cone cut appears when the central beam misses a portion of the radiographic film. The portion that is missed or does not receive radiation appears clear.

18. Which of these indicates that the radiograph was overexposed?

    c. dark image – An overexposed image will appear dark in appearance.

19. Which of these indicates that the film was not properly washed?

    c. brownish-yellow – A brownish or yellowish coloring on the exposed film indicates that either all the fixer or developer was not removed and washing was incomplete.

20. Which of these is not a cause of fogging of the radiograph?

    c. overexposure – This usually does not cause film fog but does cause darkening of processed film.

21. What is the probable cause of reticulation?

   **c. differences in processing solution temperatures –
   This will cause a "cracking" appearance, which is
   referred to as reticulation. If developer is too hot
   and fixer to cold or vice versa, reticulation can
   occur.**

22. How will static electricity appear radiographically?

   **a. as black lines – usually in the shape of a bolt of
   lightning. Static electricity can happen when a
   Panorex film is removed from the sleeve quickly
   during processing.**

23. Which of these items appears radiolucent?

   **b. dental pulp – Dental pulp will appear radiolucent
   or dark.**

24. Why would a film appear blank?

   **b. It was not exposed to radiation. – Film that
   has not been exposed to radiation will appear
   clear.**

25. Which type of crystals are embedded in the emulsion on
the film that affect the speed or sensitivity of the film?

   a. halide

26. If a patient refuses radiographs, the best course of
action would be for the office to what?

   **d. After counseling the patient and still they refuse,
   excuse the patient from practice.**

27. The lead foil found within the film packet is designed to
accomplish what function?

   **a. It is used to absorb some of the radiation that
   passes through the film and helps prevent scatter
   of radiation to the surrounding tissue.**

28. According to ANSI, which film would be considered
the fastest speed?

   d. E

29. Using a long cone will produce exposures that

   **b. are less sharp than film exposed using a short
   cone.**

30. When taking digital radiographs, the BEST way to
minimize the potential for patient cross-contamination
of the computer keyboard and mouse is to

   **b. adequately cover all surfaces with plastic
   barriers that will be contacted with gloved or
   contaminated hands.**

31. The best infection control for digital sensors is to

   **d. wipe clean with a hospital-grade disinfectant with
   no more than 80% ethanol.**

32. Which of these terms describes the ability to read
radiograph?

   **d. interpretation – To interpret a radiograph
   means the operator is able to read it and make a
   diagnosis from it.**

33. Which of these is a facial landmark?

   c. tragus

34. Which of these is not a mandibular landmark?

   a. incisive foramen

35. Which of these structures appears radiolucent?

   b. dental pulp

36. Which of these structures appears radiopaque?

   c. maxillary tuberosity

37. Which of these appears most radiopaque?

   d. enamel

38. A bony projection that extends downward and slightly
posterior in many maxillary molar radiographs is the

   d. hamular process.

39. In a radiograph of the maxillary molars, the following
structure may obscure the roots of the teeth:

   a. zygomatic process of the maxilla

40. Most dental schools now teach that for viewing,
radiographs should be mounted as though

   b. you are facing the patient.

41. Which of these helps determine whether the radiograph
is of the patient's right or left side?

   **d. identification dot – The dot on the radiograph
   tells you whether the radiograph is the patient's
   right or left side as well as whether you are
   viewing the radiograph facing the patient or
   behind the patient.**

42. When new radiographs are taken, the previous
radiographs are

   **c. placed in a coin envelope, labeled, and kept in the
   patient file – Never discard or destroy original
   radiographs or give them to anyone, including
   the patient or an insurance company.**

43. Whom do the original radiographs belong to?

   **b. the office – Contrary to popular belief,
   radiographs do not belong to the patient; they
   belong to the office. However, the patient has
   every right to a copy of those radiographs upon
   submitting a signed request.**

44. A patient is entitled to a copy of their radiographs

   **c. upon request – Contrary to popular belief, legally,
   a patient has a right to a copy of their radiographs
   no matter if they have a zero balance or not.**

45. Which item appears radiolucent on a radiograph?

   **b. periapical abscess – This will appear as a circular
   artifact just below the apex of the root of the tooth.**

46. When mounting radiographs, the dot convex tells the
evaluator that

   **b. they are viewing the patient's dentition from the
   front of the patient (facing the patient).**

47. A radiolucent mandibular landmark that can be seen around the first and second bicuspid is

    a. the mental foramen – the exit point of the mental nerve. This is a common site for anesthetizing the lower mandibular bicuspid area.

48. The pulp of the tooth on a radiograph appears

    b. radiolucent – Located in the center of the tooth, this is where the blood and nerve supply of the tooth are located.

49. The doughnut-shaped bony crests on the lingual surface of the mandible are referred to as

    b. genial tubercles – Located on the mandible below the lower central incisors, genial tubercles are used to attach muscle to the floor of the mouth.

50. The V-shaped projection from the floor of the nasal fossa in the midline is referred to as the

    c. anterior nasal spine.

51. Legal reasons radiographs should be taken may include

    d. all of the above – Diagnostic purposes, insurance records, and to compare past restorative techniques on a tooth are all reasons radiographs should be taken.

52. At the minimum, by law, the following items should appear on a radiograph mount

    a. patient's name, date, and dentist's name

53. Where should materials designed to absorb primary and secondary radiation be installed?

    d. Walls, door, and ceiling

54. Which of the following film requires the least exposure time?

    c. F-speed

55. If a patient cannot hold the film or sensor in their mouth during exposure, the best way to stabilize the sensor or the film would be to do the following:

    c. Have the patient hold the sensor or film.

56. Film that has a herringbone effect after processing has what type of exposure error?

    a. Film was exposed facing backward in the patient's mouth.

57. When reading radiographs, density can be defined as

    a. the amount of light transmitted through a film.

58. In radiographic exposure, the differences between light and dark shades is known as

    a. contrast.

59. Film sizes range between 0 and 4. Which number corresponds to the occlusal film?

    d. 4 – This is the largest of the intraoral films.

60. A film that appears too dark is a result of:

    d. overexposure.

61. When exposing radiographs, blurred images are a result of

    a. tubehead or patient movement during exposure.

62. During radiographic exposure, too much vertical angulation can result in

    d. foreshortening – This is when excessive vertical angulation can cause the image to appear shorter than it really is.

63. When mounting radiographic films, the ADA recommends that you mount the dots out. Which type of view of the patient would this indicate?

    a. The patient is facing the operator.

64. A panoramic radiograph takes a recording of which areas?

    b. the entire maxilla and mandible in one picture

65. The best film to use to detect interproximal carious lesions is referred to as what?

    d. Bitewing – These radiographs show the crown of the tooth and interproximal areas but not the root.

66. If a patient presents with a possible abscess at the apex of the tooth, the best diagnostic radiograph to take for the operator to read would be which of the following radiographs?

    c. periapical

67. Films that are processed that show the teeth elongated can be remedied by moving the position indicating device (PID) in which direction?

    b. vertically

68. Film artifacts are best described as what?

    d. Any of the above

69. When referring to radiopacity on a radiographic film, you are talking about what?

    d. the lightness or clear areas of the image on the radiograph

70. Which of the following are indications for radiographs?

    d. Any of the above can be indications to take a radiograph.

71. The _____ the film or sensor stays in the patient's mouth prior to exposure, the less likely the patient is to gag.

    b. less

72. On a periapical radiograph, what is the small circular radiolucency near the roots of the mandibular premolars?

    b. mental foramen – This landmark is visible on an x-ray and is where nerve and blood supply pass through.

73. After processing a film, it comes out clear. This could be from which error?

    c. Film was not exposed to radiation.

74. A cone cut is a result of which exposure error?

   d. **primary beam not being aimed at the center of the film**

73. When positioning a patient for a panoramic radiograph, the following should be removed:

   d. **any or all of the above – Earrings, partials or dentures, and eyewear can be seen on an x-ray as artifacts.**

74. An amalgam restoration will appear as what type of image?

   b. **radiopaque**

75. Fogged dental radiography film can be caused by what?

   d. **any of the above – Exposure to heat or light or outdated film can all cause film fog.**

76. Radiographic technique for exposing the edentulous survey requires which of the following?

   d. **Any of the above can be used when exposing radiographs on the edentulous patient.**

77. The number of exposures that comprise an adult full-mouth series is considered to be how many exposures?

   a. **18–20 exposures – A full series of radiographs usually contain four bitewings, eight posterior periapicals, and six anterior periapicals.**

78. When processing, a film that appears too dark is a result of what error occurring?

   b. **overexposure**

79. The advantage of increasing the target-film distance for patient protection is that it serves to accomplish what action?

   d. **It doesn't accomplish any of the above. – The advantage to increasing target-film distance is that it will give you a sharper and more defined radiograph.**

82. The function of an intensifying screen is designed to accomplish which task?

   d. **It is the two screens that appear on each side of the film and is used to intensify the action of the x-rays to decrease exposure to the patient.**

83. Extraoral film are utilized for which purpose?

   d. **An extraoral film can be used for any of the above reasons – extraoral film is used outside the mouth.**

84. After processing a film, you notice a lightning-bolt effect on the film. This is caused by what?

   a. **static electricity – Occasionally, when a panoramic radiograph is removed quickly from its packaging, static electricity will cause the processed film to reveal a lightning-bolt effect on the processed film.**

85. The dark areas of the radiograph are referred to as what?

   b. **radiolucent**

86. What is the best way to place film or a sensor on a patient who has mandibular tori?

   c. **between the torus and the tongue**

87. A latent image can best be described as what?

   a. **an unseen image that is on the film from exposure time until the image is processed**

88. Detail of radiographs can be best described as what?

   a. **varying degrees of shades of gray present in the image**

89. A cephalometric radiograph is primarily used for which specialty?

   c. **oral surgery due to the ability to diagnose cysts, wisdom tooth impaction, bone deformities, and other anomalies that other film will not reveal**

90. Which factor has the greatest effect on film sharpness?

   c. **kilovoltage**

91. When does distortion of an x-ray occur?

   d. **using a long target-film distance**

92. Which is most likely to produce a radiograph with long-scale contrast?

   a. **when kVp is increased**

93. The dental radiograph will appear lighter if the operator increases which setting?

   d. **film distance**

94. What is the purpose of the lead foil in the x-ray film packet?

   b. **absorb the backscatter radiation**

95. Which film is placed outside the mouth during an x-ray exposure?

   d. **Extraoral film is placed "extra" orally or outside the mouth for exposure.**

96. Which of these films uses the shortest exposure time?

   b. **screen film**

97. Which type of film is used to copy a radiograph?

   a. **duplicating film**

98. Which term best describes the process by which the latent image becomes visible?

   c. **sensitivity**

99. Which term describes a fully processed radiograph that shows a network of cracks on its surface?

   b. **reticulated**

99. A panoramic radiograph is of little value when diagnosing which condition?

   b. **recurrent caries – It is not impossible, but it is difficult to see carious lesions on a panoramic radiograph.**

100. Replenisher is added to the developing solution to accomplish what?

    d. Addition of developing solution can be added to accomplish any of the above.

101. The processing tank should be cleaned at what intervals?

    b. once a week

102. Which of the following appears more radiopaque?

    d. Amalgam will appear white or clear, which is also called radiopaque.

103. Which of these items helps determine whether an exposed radiographic image is on the patient's left or right?

    d. identification dot

104. Caries or decay in its first stages of existence is called what?

    c. incipient caries

105. Caries that occur under a restoration or around the margin of an existing crown is referred to as which type of decay?

    a. Recurrent caries are caries that were there, removed, and repaired, but redecay around the restoration occurs.

106. Which of these materials appears most radiolucent on a radiograph?

    d. Acrylic resin appears dark or radiolucent.

107. A Rinn film holder is helpful in avoiding which radiographic exposure mistake?

    d. Any of the above can be avoided using a Rinn holder.

109. In radiography, a partial shadow or fuzzy outline around the image is referred to as what?

    a. penumbra – This is the fuzziness that occurs around the image on an x-ray.

Section II:
Quality Assurance and Radiology Regulations

This section of the Radiation Health and Safety component of the Certified Dental Assisting Examination consists of 21% or 21 of the 100 multiple-choice items. The questions related to this section of the examination are based upon your knowledge of the following:

- Quality assurance
- Radiation regulations

Key Terms

EPA – Environmental Protection Agency – a regulatory agency involved in the safety and effectiveness of disinfecting and sterilizing solutions

Hazard Communication Standard – protocols established for the safe handling and disposal of chemicals in the workplace

OSHA – Occupational Safety and Health Association – a regulating body that enforces the requirements established for employers to protect their employees

safelight – a light in the red-orange spectrum that is used in darkrooms to ensure radiographs are not exposed to white light before processing

shelf life – the period of time a product can be stored and maintain its usefulness

Quick Review Outline

A. Quality Assurance

1. Evaluate film storage area

    a. Unprocessed film should be stored at 55 degrees F. It should be kept dry and free from humidity over 50%.

    b. Exposed unprocessed film should be processed as soon as possible and placed in a container away from unprocessed film or areas where radiation exposure may occur.

2. The dental assistant should possess basic knowledge regarding the storage of dental film and be able to readily identify and correct errors related to improperly storing unexposed radiographic film.

    a. All dental films are extremely sensitive to heat, humidity, pressure, and stray radiation.

        i. Heat and humidity will cause film to fog. Film should be stored in a cool, dry place. Ideally, film should be stored at 50 to 70 degrees F and 30 to 50% relative humidity.

        ii. Pressure can fog film. Do not stack film too high, and do not place heavy objects on top of the film.

        iii. Stray radiation can fog film. Film should be stored in areas shielded from radiation exposure.

    b. Dental film has a **shelf life**. The expiration date is printed on the film box, and all film should be rotated and stored where the expiration date is easily seen.

3. The assistant should understand how to prepare, maintain, and replenish radiographic solutions for manual and automatic processors.

    a. Maintenance of automatic processors requires weekly cleaning and daily checking and replenishing of solutions.

4. Identify optimum conditions for film processing

    a. Proper developer temperature should be 68 degrees F for 5 minutes.

    b. Proper fixing temperature should be between 68 and 72 degrees F. Fixing temperature is not as critical as developer temperature.

    c. The water bath should not exceed 15 degrees F difference between the developer and/or fixer to avoid reticulation.

d. All white light must be eliminated from a darkroom. It is important that there are no light leaks from around doors, fans, and vents. **Safelights** must be used when the film packets are opened, when attaching the film to the racks, and during processing procedures. A safelight will not affect the film emulsion because it is in the red-orange spectrum. Safelight filters must be free of scratches and fit precisely. The safety lights should be mounted at least 4 feet from the counter surface where the films are unwrapped. A 15-watt incandescent bulb should be used. If the safelight must be mounted closer to the counter, a lower-watt bulb, such as 7.5 watts, should used. When using indirect lighting (facing the light toward the ceiling), a 25-watt bulb may be used with the proper filters.

5. The dental assistant should understand how to implement quality-assurance procedures.

  a. daily recording of solution temperatures

  b. dates of solution changes

  c. test film runs

  d. cleaning and maintaining equipment

  e. periodic inspections

  f. Other quality-assurance tests may include the step-wedge technique. This technique measures the quality of the processing solutions. Other techniques like the coin test can be implemented to check for darkroom light leaks.

B. Radiology Regulations

1. The dental assistant should be familiar with preparing radiographs for legal requirements, viewing, and duplication.

  a. The dental assistant should be able to identify methods for duplicating radiographs.

    i. Duplicating radiographs is usually done in the darkroom using a duplicator and duplicating film. The film is processed as usual. Duplicating digital radiographs requires the assistant to be able to use the computer software program to copy radiographs into other applications throughout the patient's chart or the ability to copy the radiograph and/or email it to the appropriate requesting office.

  b. The dental assistant should be able to identify information that must legally appear on the mount label.

    i. At the minimum, the patient's name, date the radiograph was taken, and the dental office it was taken at should appear on the mount or patient record if you are taking digital radiographs. Some offices put the patient's chart number, age or birthdate, and, area of interest (i.e., tooth #4).

  c. The dental assistant should be able to identify reasons for exposing and retaining radiographs.

    i. Some reasons the assistant may offer for exposing and retaining radiographs may include legal reasons, insurance requires the radiograph be submitted to pay a claim, diagnostic purposes, and possible need for future reference.

    ii. A patient can legally obtain a copy of the radiographs taken at the dental office at any time. Normally, the originals are maintained by the office, but copies should always be presented when requested. A patient must sign a waiver to release these radiographs if they are going to another dental office. If they are being used for legal purposes, a subpoena by the patient's attorney will suffice.

    iii. Some states allow the dental office to charge a fee for this duplication, but most offices will perform this free of charge.

    iv. Often, a patient will request a set to be emailed, and this is acceptable as well, but a release should still be obtained or some notation in the patient's chart made indicating who the radiographs were sent to.

    v. Permission from a patient does not have to be obtained when radiographs are sent to an insurance company in order to process a claim.

2. The dental assistant should be familiar with the proper storage of chemical agents used in radiography procedures according to the local regulatory agency, in compliance with the **OSHA Hazard Communication Standard**. Each state has its own regulatory procedures for storage and disposal of radiography chemicals.

3. The dental assistant should be able to describe how to properly dispose of all chemical agents and other materials used in dental radiography procedures.

   a. Developer and water may be placed down the sink with water. However, fixer, since it contains silver salts, must be kept in a labeled plastic container and picked up by a licensed hauler. The **Environmental Protection Agency (EPA)** expects maintained logs reflecting the disposal of fixer to be available for inspection.

Important Objectives to Know

- Preparing, maintaining, and replenishing radiographic solutions for manual and automatic processors
- Properly disposing of all chemical agents and other materials used in dental radiography procedures
- Implementing quality-assurance procedures such as solution maintenance, test film runs, cleaning and maintaining the equipment, and record of periodic inspections
- Identify optimum conditions and procedures for processing radiographs.
- Know how to properly store chemical agents used in radiography procedures according to the local regulatory agency and the compliance of all OSHA Hazard Communication Standards.
- Preparing radiographs for legal requirements
- Identifying methods for duplicating radiographs
- Identifying information that must legally appear on the radiograph mount
- Know the proper method for storing radiographs.

Study Checklist

1. Review your textbook information on processing radiographs.
2. Review all terminology related to processing radiographs.
3. Review CDC and OSHA guidelines as they relate to radiograph processing.
5. Understand information as it relates to all radiographic processing chemicals.

Section II:
Quality Assurance and Radiology Regulations – Review Questions

Use the Answer Sheet found in Appendix A.

1. According to the EPA, spent fixer chemicals should be disposed of in the following manner:
   a. sent down the lab sink following three minutes of hot water.
   b. picked up by a licensed hauler.
   c. placed in a spillproof container and stored for future disposal in the office.
   d. placed in a punctureproof container and placed in the regular trash.

2. The drifting of the tubehead should only be corrected by
   a. the dental assistant.
   b. the dentist.
   c. a trained repair person.
   d. the salesman who sold the equipment to your office.

3. Automatic processors require
   a. minimal servicing.
   b. weekly cleaning and chemical change.
   c. monthly chemical change.
   d. daily maintenance.

4. Regardless of who exposes and processes the radiographs, the final responsibility rests with
   a. the dentist.
   b. the office manager.
   c. the dental assistant.
   d. the radiography equipment manufacturer.

5. Which testing device is used in quality control to compare the density of the radiographic image?
   a. a safelight
   b. a step wedge
   c. a viewer
   d. a photoreceptor

6. Processing solutions should be changed about every
   a. day.
   b. week.
   c. 1 to 2 weeks.
   d. 4 weeks.

7. What happens to the radiograph when a film is exposed to a safelight too long?
   a. The radiograph appears white.
   b. The radiograph appears fogged.
   c. The radiograph becomes reticulated.
   d. The radiograph appears with dark spots.

8. Which term best describes the process by which the latent image becomes visible?
   a. reticulation
   b. reduction

c. sensitivity
d. preservation

9. How far above the work area in the darkroom should the safelight be located?
   a. 6–8 inches
   b. 1½ feet
   c. 2½ feet
   d. 4 feet

10. Which of these is the correct processing sequence?
    a. rinse, fix, wash, develop, dry
    b. fix, rinse, develop, wash, dry
    c. develop, rinse, fix, wash, dry
    d. rinse, develop, wash, fix, dry

11. Which of the following reduces the exposed silver bromide crystals?
    a. developer
    b. wetting agent
    c. fixer
    d. cutting

12. Which ingredient of the developer is alkaline and causes the emulsion to soften and swell?
    a. the developing agent
    b. the preservative
    c. the activator
    d. the restrainer

13. Which developing chemical becomes extremely active when the temperature is raised?
    a. sodium sulfite
    b. potassium bromide
    c. elon
    d. hydroquinone

14. Which ingredient of the fixer removes all unexposed and any remaining undeveloped silver halide crystals?
    a. the fixing agent
    b. the preservative
    c. the activator
    d. the restrainer

15. The film emulsion is hardened during
    a. development.
    b. rinsing.
    c. fixation.
    d. washing.

16. The floating thermometer for manual processing should be placed in the
    a. developing solution.
    b. water compartment.
    c. fixing solution.
    d. both B and C.

17. Light leaks in the darkroom will cause
    a. lightening of the film.
    b. film fog.
    c. underdeveloped film.
    d. underexposed film.

18. The processing tank should be cleaned
    a. every day.
    b. once a week.
    c. every 2 weeks.
    d. whenever the solutions are changed.

19. What is the ideal temperature when film is processed manually?
    a. 60 degrees F
    b. 68 degrees F
    c. 75 degrees F
    d. 83 degrees F

20. Chemically, what is the major difference between solutions used for manual processing and those used for rapid and automatic processing?
    a. There is more acid in rapid-processing solution.
    b. Manual processing solutions contain more preservatives.
    c. Rapid and automatic processing solutions contain more hardener.
    d. Manual processing solutions are more alkaline.

21. Replenisher is added to the developing solution to
    a. compensate for oxidation.
    b. compensate for loss of volume.
    c. compensate for loss of solution strength.
    d. all of the above.

22. If a patient needs their radiographs transferred to another office, the best way to accomplish this is by
    a. giving the patient their original set if they have a zero balance.
    b. letting the patient borrow them for their new appointment a the new office.
    c. having the patient sign a release, giving the patient a copy, and keeping the original in the office.
    d. retaking another set and giving that set to the patient.

23. Stirring rods or paddles are utilized during darkroom processing for which purpose?
    a. agitating the rinse
    b. mixing the developer and fixer
    c. obtaining uniform concentration throughout the solutions
    d. The stirring rods and paddles can be utilized for any of the above items.

24. The fixing agent used in processing radiographs accomplishes which objective?
    a. hardens the emulsion
    b. prevents further development
    c. removes unexposed silver bromide crystals
    d. reduces the rate of oxidation

25. Which is the best way to discard radiographic fixer?
    a. Pour it down the drain along with hot water.
    b. Store it in a container and then dispose of it in the regular garbage.
    c. Have it hauled away by a licensed hauler.
    d. Mix it with the developer to deactivate it and pour it down the sink.

26. The design of the darkroom should be light leakproof for what reason?
    a. prevent underexposure
    b. prevent a clear film from occurring
    c. prevent fogged or black film
    d. prevent contamination

27. Optimal developing time for an automatic or manual processing tank should be in which temperature range?
    a. 55–58 degrees F
    b. 60–65 degrees F
    c. 68–70 degrees F
    d. 75–80 degrees F

28. The purpose of the darkroom film developer is to react with what product to produce an image?
    a. ammonium thiosulfate
    b. silver halide crystals
    c. hydrobromide
    d. chlorinated ions

29. What happens to a film when the safelight does not contain the appropriate bulb/filter?
    a. The radiograph appears white.
    b. The radiograph appears fogged.
    c. The radiograph becomes reticulated.
    d. The radiograph becomes too dark.

30. How far above the work area in the darkroom should the safelight be located?
    a. 6–8 inches
    b. 1.5 feet
    c. 2.5 feet
    d. 4 feet

31. Which of these is the correct sequence for radiographic film processing?
    a. rinse, fix, wash, develop, and dry
    b. fix, rinse, develop, wash, and dry
    c. develop, rinse, fix, wash, and dry
    d. rinse, develop, wash, fix, and dry

32. The floating thermometer for manual processing should be placed in which solution?
    a. developer
    b. fixer
    c. water
    d. either b or c

33. Light leaks in the darkroom will cause which of the following to occur?
    a. lightening of the film
    b. film fog
    c. underdeveloped film
    d. underexposed film

Section II:
Quality Assurance and Radiology Regulations – Answers and Rationales

1. According to the EPA, spent fixer chemicals should be disposed of in the following manner:

   b. picked up by a licensed hauler – Spent or exhausted fixer can only be disposed of by a licensed hauler. That means that someone with the proper licensing to dispose of hazardous waste must come to your place of business and pick it up.

2. The drifting of the tubehead should only be corrected by

   a. the dental assistant – This repair does not have to be done by a trained repairperson as most often the cause is just a loose screw or fitting and can be either tightened or replaced by an employee who has basic knowledge of the unit. If the problem goes beyond the scope or knowledge of the employee, only then do you have to call in a repair person.

3. Automatic processors require

   b. automatic processors require very minimal servicing, however, daily monitoring of chemical and water levels, weekly replenishing and cleaning of the inside moving parts, and maintenance or repair is required.

4. Regardless of who exposes and processes the radiographs, the final responsibility rests with

   a. the dentist – The dentist is responsible for making a diagnosis from radiographs, and ultimately, she or he should have examined each and every radiograph that is taken in the office for both quality and diagnostic purposes.

5. Which testing device is used in quality control to compare the density of the radiographic image?

   b. a step wedge – This device consists of increments of absorber through which a radiographic exposure is made on film to permit determination of the amounts of radiation reaching the film by measurements density.

6. Processing solutions should be changed about every

   b. week – Usually once a week is sufficient for chemical usage. Chemical exhaustion usually occurs after one week unless the processor is used at an usually high rate.

7. happens to the radiograph when a film is exposed to a safelight too long?

   b. The radiograph appears fogged. – The radiograph will appear fogged or hazy if the safelight has been exposed to it for too long.

8. Which term best describes the process by which the latent image becomes visible?

   c. sensitivity – The coating on the radiographic film is a gelatinous solution containing silver halides. Sensitivity of the film to radiation exposure describes the process by which the latent image becomes visible.

9. How far above the work area in the darkroom should the safelight be located?

   d. 4 feet – This is the ideal distance the safelight should be located from the work area.

10. Which of these is the correct processing sequence?

    c. develop, rinse, fix, wash, dry – Developing, rinsing, fixing, washing, and then drying is the proper sequence. A film does not have to be rinsed prior to developing.

11. Which of the following reduces the exposed silver bromide crystals?

    a. developer – the activator in the developing solution exposes silver bromide crystals.

12. Which ingredient of the developer is alkaline and causes the emulsion to soften and swell?

    c. the activator – This product in the developer lets more of the exposed silver bromide crystals come into contact with the developing agents.

13. Which developing chemical becomes extremely active when the temperature is raised?

    d. hydroquinone – While most chemicals are accelerated by heat, hydroquinone is extremely active at higher temperatures.

14. Which ingredient of the fixer removes all unexposed and any remaining undeveloped silver halide crystals?

    a. the fixing agent – This will stop further development.

15. The film emulsion is hardened during

    c. fixation – This is the stage when the film emulsion is hardened.

16. The floating thermometer for manual processing should be placed in the

    a. developing solution – Since developing solutions are the most sensitive to temperature, a thermometer should be used in the developing tank.

17. Light leaks in the darkroom will cause

    b. film fog – Film fog can be caused by light leak or overexposure of safelight, so by closing the door and shutting the lights off, you are able to see any light leaks present and correct them to prevent fogging.

18. The processing tank should be cleaned

    b. once a week – When changing exhausted chemicals, cleaning the entire processing tank should be done as well.

19. What is the ideal temperature when film is processed manually?

    b. 68 degrees F

20. Chemically, what is the major difference between solutions used for manual processing and those used for rapid and automatic processing?

    c. Rapid and automatic processing solutions contain more hardener. – This hardening agent is added to facilitate the transportation of the films through the roller systems of the automatic units.

21. Replenisher is added to the developing solution to

    d. all of the above – Oxidation, volume, and solution strength are all valid reasons for replenishing developer and fixer.

22. If a patient needs their radiographs transferred to another office, the best way to accomplish this is by

    c. having the patient sign a release, giving the patient a copy, and keeping the original in the office.

23. Stirring rods or paddles are utilized during darkroom processing for which purpose?

    d. The stirring rods and paddles can be utilized for any of the above items.

24. The fixing agent used in processing radiographs accomplishes which objective?

    c. removes unexposed silver bromide crystals

25. Which is the best way to discard radiographic fixer?

    c. Have it hauled away by a licensed hauler. – Fixer contains silver salts and should never be discarded down the drain as it can contaminate ground water supply.

26. The design of the darkroom should be light leakproof for what reason?

    c. prevent fogged or black film

27. Optimal developing time for an automatic or manual processing tank should be in which temperature range?

    b. 60–65 degrees F

28. The purpose of the darkroom film developer is to react with what product to produce an image?

    b. silver halide crystals

29. What happens to a film when it is exposed to the safelight too long?

    d. The radiograph appears dark.

30. How far above the work area in the darkroom should the safelight be located?

    d. 4 feet

31. Which of these is the correct sequence for radiographic film processing?

    c. develop, rinse, fix, wash, and dry

32. The floating thermometer for manual processing should be placed in which solution?

    a. developer

33. Light leaks in the darkroom will cause which of the following to occur?

    b. film fog

Section III:
Radiation Safety for Patients and Operators

This section of the Radiation Health and Safety component of the Certified Dental Assisting Examination consists of 31% or 31 of the 100 multiple-choice items. The questions related to this section of the examination are based upon your knowledge of the following:

- Identify current ADA guidelines for frequency of exposure to radiation.
- Physics and the principles of radiation protection when operating radiographic equipment
- Be able to practice patient safety measures to provide protection from x-radiation.
- Address patient concerns about radiation, including informed consent or patient refusals of radiography.
- Demonstrate an understanding of operator safety measures to provide protection from radiation.
- Describe techniques for monitoring individual exposure to radiation.

Key Terms

ALARA – the principle of keeping radiation exposure "as low as reasonably achievable"; it involves combining radiation protection procedures with commonsense practices

atom – smallest particle of a substance

collimator – a device used to eliminate peripheral radiation

composition of matter – substances that make up a particular material

fast film – refers to the speed of film; fast film requires lower amounts of exposure time

film badge – a device worn to detect levels of radiation exposure

filter – a device used to eliminate x-rays outside the useful range of exposure

filtration – the ability to distinguish and remove that which is not useful for diagnostic radiation

ionization – process by which atoms change into negatively or positively charged ions during radiation

lead apron – device used to block radiation exposure to sensitive tissues

maximum permissible dose – the maximum dose of radiation that, in light of present knowledge, would not be expected to produce negative effects in a life

pocket dosimeter – a device worn to detect levels of radiation exposure

position indicating device (PID) – the open-ended tube in a dental x-ray unit, commonly called the cone

primary beam – central beam of the x-ray tubehead

scatter radiation – radiation that is deflected from its path as it strikes matter

secondary radiation – formed when the primary x-rays strike the patient or come in contact with any matter or substance

x-ray – invisible, odorless electromagnetic radiation

Quick Review Outline

A. The dental assistant should be able to identify the ADA guidelines for determining frequency of exposure.
   1. The dental assistant to should pay close attention to the patient's overall exposure potential. If the patient has recently undergone radiation therapy, dental radiographs should be minimized. Also, taking radiographs just because "the patient is due" is not a reason to take radiographs. Some patients require radiographs more often than others, and by the same token, some patients do not require radiographs as often as others.

B. Apply the principles of radiation protection and health physics and hazards in the operation of radiographic equipment. Radiation protection is key for both the operator and the patient. A complete understanding of the effects of radiation exposure on humans should be understood by the dental assistant. Knowing how to properly set up and operate the radiography machine and realizing the potential effects of exposure are key in practicing radiation safety.

1. Identify the factors affecting x-ray production, including kVp, mA, and exposure time.

   a. Kilovoltage peak (kVp) is the measurement of electromotive force, equal to 1000 volts. High kilovoltage is essential for the production of dental x-rays. This measurement determines the penetration power of x-rays that are emitted. The kVp setting is one of the most important factors that determines the image contrast, as well as dosage to the patient.

   b. Milliamperage (mA) is defined as 1000th of an ampere. In radiography, the milliamperage determines the number of electrons available at the filament. Milliamperage determines the quantity (amount) of x-rays that are emitted from the tubehead of the x-ray machine.

   c. Exposure time is defined as the amount of time an area is bombarded with radiation emission. Duration of time is directly related to kVP and milliamperage. Density of tissue and areas exposed are also considered factors.

2. The dental assistant should be able to describe the characteristics of radiation. Some of these characteristics may include density, contrast, kilovoltage, milliamperage, and intensity.

3. The dental assistant should be able to demonstrate an understanding of x-ray machine factors that influence radiation safety, including concepts of filtration, shielding, collimation, and PID (cone) length.

   a. **Filtration** is described as the filtering of less-desirable x-rays during the exposure process using an aluminum **filter**. These less-desirable x-rays decrease the patient's overall exposure and are not generally helpful in the final quality of the radiograph.

   b. Shielding is a concept used in the dental office that applies to the protection of either the operator or the patient. Operator shielding includes lead-lined walls and placing yourself outside the **primary beam**. In today's offices, shielding is rarely needed because of the use of **fast film** and small beam diameter. However, precautions are still followed by requiring the operator to stand at a 135-degree angle to the patient, at least 6 feet away from the patient, and out of the path of the primary beam. Most dental offices have gypsum or drywall, and this provides an adequate barrier for the other patients or operators not involved in exposing radiographs. Dental radiographs are safe and generally do not pose a health risk when the patient is wearing proper protection such as lead-lined aprons with thyroid coverage that are designed to protect the patient's torso, including the reproductive area.

   c. Collimation, when used properly, serves to limit the size and shape of the useful x-ray beam reaching the patient. This not only reduces the dose, but it also improves image quality. The ADA recommends a rectangular **collimator**, but round collimators are more commonly found. The restriction of the useful beam to an appropriate size is generally to a diameter of 2¼ in. (7 cm) at the skin surface.

   d. **Position indicating device (PID)** or cone length is referred to as the cylindrical cone that indicates the direction of the central beam of radiation. The length of the cone helps establish the desired target-surface distance. The PID guides the primary beam target.

4. The dental assistant should be able to demonstrate an understanding of x-radiation physics such as primary radiation and scatter (secondary) radiation (Figure 2-27).

   a. Primary radiation is the radiation that is the original undeflected useful beam of radiation that emanates at the focal spot of the x-ray tube and emerges though the aperture of the tubehead. This is the main beam of radiation emitted from the x-ray unit.

   b. **Scatter (secondary) radiation** is given off by any matter irradiated with x-rays. This form of radiation is created at the instant the primary beam interacts with matter and gives off some of its energy, forming new and less powerful wavelengths. This type of radiation is also referred to as "scatter" radiation.

5. The dental assistant should be able to explain the protocol for suspected x-ray machine malfunctions.

   a. X-ray machine malfunctions can occur and are usually detected only after quality radiographs are not obtained. Many malfunctions can be avoided by following simple steps to ensure that the radiography equipment is working at peak performance. The following testing can be performed by licensed technicians or dental practitioners. The following test tests should be performed annually.

      i. x-ray output
      ii. kilovoltage calibration

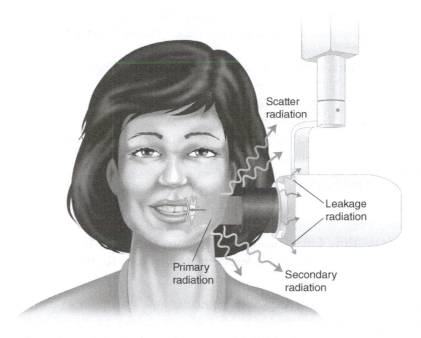

Figure 2-27 Primary, secondary, and leakage radiation identified on an x-ray tube and patient's face.

      iii. half value layer
      iv. timer accuracy
       v. milliamperage output
      vi. collimation
     vii. beam alignment
    viii. tubehead stability

C. Practice patient safety measures

1. The dental assistant should be able to identify major causes of unnecessary x-radiation exposure. One of the biggest causes of unnecessary x-radiation is exposure. Taking radiographs because "the patient is due" is not a good reason. When there is no real need, there should be no exposure. Dentists should follow reasonable guidelines when prescribing radiographs. For example, adolescents would be likely to have radiographs more often than middle-aged adults who rarely have restorative procedures performed.

2. The dental assistant should be able to demonstrate an understanding of x-radiation biology with regard to short- and long-term effects of x-radiation on cells and tissues and effective doses.

   a. Routine radiographs rarely produce any permanent cellular damage. However, when radiation is used in oral cancer treatment, the patient can suffer from cell and tissue damage, mucosal inflammation, decrease in salivary flow, and permanent tissue damage.

   b. Short-term effects of ionizing radiation include redness around the area irradiated.

   c. Long-term effects of ionizing radiation can cause tissue death or permanent damage.

   d. Biological effects begin with the ionization of atoms. This mechanism causes damage to human tissue. When ionizing radiation interacts with cells, it may or may not strike a critical part of the cell. Chromosomes are the most critical part of the cell, and since they contain genetic information and instructions required for the cell to perform its function and copy itself, if this part of the cell is damaged, it ceases to multiply or multiplies into a mutated cell.

   e. Possible effects of radiation on cells include no damage, damaged cells that still operate, cells that are damaged, cells that repair the damage and operate abnormally, and actual cell death. The effects that appear in a matter of minutes, days, or weeks are called acute effects. During these exposures, an event that generally follows is known as a dose-response period, meaning the response of the tissue from the dose of radiation.

f. All cells are not equally sensitive to radiation damage. In general, cells that divide rapidly, such as bone marrow, tend to show effects at lower doses of radiation than those that are less rapidly dividing and more specialized, like skin.

g. The dental assistant should be able to demonstrate an understanding of the concepts of both an x-radiation dose and effective dose, which is the dose that accounts for different radiosensitivities of different tissues.

3. The dental assistant should be able to identify ways to reduce x-radiation exposure to patients (**ALARA**) and guidelines that determine frequency of exposure. ALARA stands for "as low as reasonably achievable" and means that the goal of the dental office is to obtain diagnostic information while keeping the exposure to the patient and dental staff at minimum levels.

a. The most commonly used mode of protection for the patient is the **lead apron**. The lead apron covers the entire chest and lap, effectively reducing scatter radiation reaching underlying tissues. Lead aprons come either with the thyroid collar attached or as a separate apron and collar.

b. Film speed is also a consideration in patient safety. Film speed ranges from A to F. The farther down the alphabet, the faster the film, which means less exposure. Groups D, E, and F are the most commonly used in the dental field. Digital radiographs have eliminated the need for film speed.

D. Address patient concerns about radiation

1. Explain to your patient that radiation exposure, no matter how small, carries with it some risk. We know, that on average, these risks are comparable to or smaller than risks we encounter in other activities or occupations we consider safe. So we adhere to the ALARA principle, keep equipment tested, and protect the patient with barriers. Also, the diagnostic benefit of dental radiographs far outweighs the risks and are needed for accurate diagnosis and patient care. Genetic mutations can appear in future generations, however, when reproductive cells of the individual irradiated are damaged.

E. The dental assistant must demonstrate understanding of operator safety measures to provide protection from radiation.

1. Identify sources of radiation to operators and other staff while exposing images.

2. Identify safety measures to reduce operator exposure to radiation.

b. Safety measures that provide protection from overexposure to x-radiation include:

   i. personal monitoring devices

   ii. observe the **maximum permissible** dose of 5 rems per year

   iii. Equipment that ensures minimum exposure, such as a shorter position indicating device, decreases exposure to both dental healthcare worker and patient.

   iv. **film badge**: A film badge is worn by the operator and is turned into a monitoring company that will test the badge for exposure. Results are sent back to the office. If the operator is receiving too much exposure, equipment is tested and adjusted. If the operator is receiving an exposure amount in compliance within the standards of exposure, no action is taken.

   v. The operator is required to stand at least 6 feet from the head of the patient. This gives an appropriate and safe distance during exposure.

   vi. For safety reasons, the operator must stay out of the path of the primary beam.

   vii. Never hold the film for the patient. Holding the film for a patient during exposure repeatedly exposes the dental healthcare worker to unnecessary radiation.

   viii. Never hold the tubehead during exposure.

   ix. Always use the fastest film speed possible to decrease exposure times.

   x. Lead-lined walls, which are rarely used in the dental office, or walls made of gypsum give adequate protection for the operator and other members of the team.

3. Demonstrate an understanding of terms related to radiation physics and biology pertaining to operator exposure.

a. Basic terms the dental assistant should be familiar with:

    i. **Composition of matter** includes all physical things that are composed of matter that are inert but occupy space. They can be gas, solid, or liquid.

    ii. **Atoms** are the fundamental units of any element and are composed of the nucleus and orbiting electrons.

    iii. **Ionization** occurs when an electrically neutral atom loses an electron. It becomes a positively charged ion and the free electron a negative ion. The process of losing or gaining an electron is known as ionization.

    iv. **Radiation** is the transmission of energy through space (or matter) and consists of electromagnetic (non-particulate) and particulate energy. Particulate energy consists of alpha rays, beta rays, cathode rays, and fast-moving electrons.

    v. An **x-ray** is an invisible beam of light, and the x-ray machine consists of a control panel and the head of the x-ray machine that contains an x-ray tube and generators that receive alternating current from the control panel.

F. The dental assistant should be aware of the various personal monitoring devices and what their functions are. These devices are worn by dental office staff members and measure how much radiation they are receiving. Monitoring devices vary in cost and effectiveness. Some devices only indicate that radiation has been received, while others show the amount and still others actually measure the amount and type of radiation. If you work around radiation, you are required to wear a monitoring device at all times while on duty. Some personal monitoring devices are listed below.

    a. **pocket dosimeter**

    b. film badge

    c. thermoluminescent dosimeter

    d. TLD badges

Important Objectives to Know

1. Understand the ionizing effects of radiation exposure to the patient.
2. Know the protocol for testing and maintaining radiograph equipment for the safety of the patient.
3. Be familiar with barriers used in the protection of the patient during exposure.
4. Understand the factors affecting x-ray production, including kVp, mA, and exposure time.
5. Be able to explain x-ray machine factors that influence radiation safety, including concepts of filtration, shielding, collimation, and PID (cone) length.
6. Understand what primary and secondary radiation is.
7. Describe protocol for suspected x-ray machine malfunctions.

Study Checklist

1. Review text information as it relates to operator safety.
2. Review all terminology related to operator safety.
3. Review any lab manual chapters as they relate to operator and staff safety.
4. Review text information as it relates to patient safety when exposing radiographs.
5. Review all terminology related to patient safety during exposing dental radiographs.
6. Review any lab manual chapters as they relate to the operation of the radiographic equipment.

Section III:
Radiation Safety for Patients and Operators –
Review Questions

Use the Answer Sheet found in Appendix A.

1. Who has the legal responsibility for all acts and services performed in the dental office?
   a. the dental hygienist
   b. the dental technician
   c. the dental assistant
   d. the dentist

2. Which of these terms best describes the x-rays that are coming directly from the focal spot on the target of the x-ray tube?
   a. filtered beam
   b. secondary beam
   c. primary beam
   d. scatter beam

3. Who is the only person who should be in the path of the primary beam?
   a. the dentist
   b. the patient
   c. the dental assistant
   d. the receptionist

4. Which item is made of aluminum?
   a. a dosimeter
   b. a filter
   c. a collimator
   d. a primary barrier

5. What material is the collimator made of?
   a. copper
   b. tungsten
   c. samarium
   d. lead

6. The purpose of the collimator is to
   a. shape the x-ray beam.
   b. remove many of the long-wavelength x-rays.
   c. increase the energy of the x-ray beam.
   d. increase scatter radiation.

7. The purpose of the filter is to
   a. shape the x-ray beam.
   b. remove many of the long-wavelength x-rays.
   c. remove many of the short-wavelength x-rays from the primary beam.
   d. prevent tubehead leakage.

8. Which of these is not an event that follows major exposure to radiation?
   a. a dose-response period
   b. a latent period
   c. a period of injury
   d. a recovery period

9. Which of these is the earliest detectable symptom of excessive radiation exposure?
   a. erythema
   b. xerostomia
   c. alopecia
   d. dysphagia

10. Which of these is not considered to be a possible long-term effect of exposure to radiation?
    a. cataracts
    b. arthritis
    c. embryological defects
    d. genetic mutations

11. Radiation injuries that do not appear in the person irradiated but occur in future generations are called
    a. long-term effects.
    b. somatic effects.
    c. genetic effects.
    d. threshold effects.

12. The earliest detectable physical change due to a large radiation exposure is
    a. shortening of the life span.
    b. sterility.
    c. presence of mutations.
    d. a drop in lymphocyte count.

13. Those effects that appear within a matter of minutes, days, or weeks are called
    a. acute effects.
    b. latent effects.
    c. long-term effects.
    d. accumulated effects.

14. The cylindrical cone that indicates the direction of the central beam of radiation is also called the
    a. PID.
    b. CMID.
    c. CID.
    d. MID.

15. Another form of radiation that is given off by any matter irradiated with x-rays is
    a. primary radiation.
    b. secondary or scatter radiation.
    c. backscatter radiation.
    d. mutating radiation.

16. Kilovoltage is best described as
    a. the measurement of electromotive force, equal to 1000 volts.
    b. 1/10th of a volt.
    c. the electrical charge of a particle.
    d. the factor that determines how clear the radiograph is.

17. When a cell is damaged by radiation,
    a. it always causes death to the cell.
    b. it may repair the damage and operate normally.
    c. it induces radiation poisoning.
    d. there is a high probability of cancer.

18. If radiation causes damage to a cell and the cell is not effectively repaired,
    a. the outcome is always cancer.
    b. any future offspring of the person will carry the mutation.
    c. the cell may be removed by the immune system.
    d. the cell will die.

19. The mechanism that cases damage to cells from radiation exposure is
    a. ionization.
    b. dispensation.
    c. reticulation.
    d. hydrolyzation.

20. Genetic effects of radiation appear in the future generation of the exposed person as a result of radiation damage to the
    a. reproductive cells.
    b. bone marrow.
    c. blood cells.
    d. brain cells.

21. Name the biggest cause of unnecessary radiation overexposure.
    a. having the kVp set too high
    b. using slow-speed film
    c. taking radiographs just because "the patient is due"
    d. taking a full-mouth series every 3 years

22. The maximum permissible dose of radiation per year for dental healthcare workers should not exceed
    a. 5 rems per year.
    b. 10 rems per year.
    c. 15 rems per year.
    d. 20 rems per year.

23. To maximize operator safety during patient exposure, the operator should
    a. stand next to the patient.
    b. stand at least 6 feet away from the patient's head.
    c. use a lead apron.
    d. use fast-speed film.

24. Which of the following is not a personal monitoring device?
    a. pocket dosimeter
    b. film badge
    c. PID device
    d. thermoluminescent dosimeter

25. The three major elements that make up the x-ray machine are
    a. the PID, the collimator, and the operating panel.
    b. the vacuum tube, the high-voltage power source, and the operating console.
    c. the tubehead, the PID, and the vacuum tube.
    d. the control panel, the high-voltage power source, and the collimator.

26. An atom is defined as
    a. the fundamental unit of any element; composed of the nucleus and orbiting electrons.
    b. one or more units of any element combined to create energy.
    c. negatively charged elements that circle the nucleus.
    d. positively charged ions released when electrical activity is applied.

27. Ionization occurs when
    a. the proton in the nucleus exchanges an electron with the neutron, which creates energy.
    b. electrons are bundled together to create more energy.
    c. a positive electron exchanges its positiveness for a proton.
    d. an electrically neutral atom loses an electron and becomes a positively charged ion and the free electron a negative ion.

28. The operating console
    a. is the control unit, which works to manage the currents, voltage, and timer.
    b. controls the position indicating device.
    c. generates the x-rays used in the exposure of dental radiographs.
    d. controls the deadman switch in exposure of x-rays.

29. Due to the energy within them, x-rays use which type of waves to break through the many layers of body tissues?
    a. heat
    b. electromagnetic
    c. radioactive
    d. electronic

30. Which of the following is not a source of radiation exposure?
    a. microwave
    b. television monitors
    c. computer monitor
    d. ultrasonic instrument cleaner

31. A film badge is
    a. worn by the operator and is turned in to a monitoring company that will test the badge for exposure.
    b. placed in the operatory to monitor radiation exposure.
    c. attached to the patient to monitor radiation exposure.
    d. always evaluated at the end of the year for exposure levels.

32. What is the purpose of a personal monitoring device?
    a. It monitors the amount of x-rays an operator takes in one 24-hour period.
    b. It monitors how much radiation is in the office.
    c. It monitors how much radiation is given off by sources other than the x-ray machine.
    d. It monitors how much radiation an individual operator is being exposed to in a given timeframe.

33. The ALARA principle, as it relates to operator safety, is followed by
    a. ensuring the operator is standing at least 6 feet from the patient.
    b. using personal monitoring devices.
    c. checking equipment often for safety and effectiveness.
    d. all of the above.

34. Ionizing radiation has the potential to produce biological damage
    a. because x-rays can detach subatomic particles from larger molecules.
    b. because they create an electrical imbalance within a normally stable cell.
    c. because they contain heat, which burns the cell and causes it to die.
    d. A and B only

35. Which term best describes radiation of natural origin?
    a. background radiation
    b. scatter radiation
    c. ionizing radiation
    d. leakage radiation

36. Which of these cells is most radiosensitive?
    a. muscle cells
    b. nerve cells
    c. red blood cells
    d. mature bone cells

37. Which of these cells is most radioresistant?
    a. red blood cells
    b. muscle cells
    c. epithelial cells
    d. white blood cells

38. Which of the tissues that can be in the path of the dental x-ray beam is most radioresistant?
    a. lens of the eye
    b. thyroid gland
    c. red bone marrow in the mandible
    d. the enamel of the teeth

39. The tissue that is most sensitive to radiation is
    a. skin.
    b. muscle.
    c. bone.
    d. lymphoid.

40. Which of these factors has no effect on determining the extent of radiation injury?
    a. the area exposed
    b. the age of the patient
    c. the type of film used
    d. the dose rate

41. Direct effects of radiation
    a. include damaging effects on a biological, cellular, or molecular level.
    b. cannot be measured.
    c. are not a concern if the patient is properly protected.
    d. are only controlled by the type of x-ray unit you use.

42. The letters ALARA stand for
    a. as low as reasonably accumulated.
    b. as latent as responsive accumulation.
    c. as low as reasonable achievable.
    d. after lower accumulation radiation aggregation.

43. What would be a common way to monitor the amount of scatter radiation a healthcare worker may be exposed to?
    a. dosimeter badge
    b. lead control device
    c. a lead ring inside the tubehead
    d. a collimator inside the tubehead

44. Where is the safest position for an operator while exposing an intraoral film?
    a. behind the patient
    b. next to the primary beam
    c. to the right of the patient
    d. at a 45-degree angle on the opposite side of the patient

45. The physical effect of radiation is
    a. incremental.
    b. varied.
    c. acute.
    d. cumulative.

46. Which of the following group of tissues can be considered the MOST sensitive to radiation exposure?
    a. kidney, muscle, and nerve tissue
    b. salivary glands, thyroid, and liver
    c. connective tissue and growing bone
    d. lymphoid, reproductive cells, and bone marrow

47. For radiation exposure, kilovotage (kV) can be best described as
    a. It controls the total time rays flow from the x-ray tube.
    b. It determines the quality of penetrating power of the central beam.
    c. It determines the amount of radiation exposure received.
    d. It determines the amount of amperes that the tubehead releases.

48. The ALARA concept emphasizes using the _____ amount of radiation exposure possible.
    a. lowest
    b. highest
    c. strongest
    d. weakest

49. What is the lead disk that is placed over the opening of the x-ray head referred to?
    a. anode disc
    b. cathode tube
    c. lead collimator
    d. diaphragm

50. Which item is used to absorb low-energy x-rays that have little penetrating power?
    a. collimator
    b. aluminum filter

c. lead washer

d. PID

51. The best way to protect the patient from radiation exposure to the reproductive and thyroid areas is to ensure what happens?

    a. use of a lead apron

    b. use of thyroid collar

    c. Have the patient sit in an upright position.

    d. Use a lead apron with thyroid collar attached.

52. To increase the penetrating quality of an x-ray beam, the auxiliary must do which of the following?

    a. increase kVp (kilovoltage peak)

    b. decrease kVp

    c. use a collimator

    d. increase the mA (milliamperage)

53. Scatter radiation is what type of radiation?

    a. secondary radiation

    b. primary radiation

    c. ambient radiation

    d. solar

54. The position indicating device (PID) can be best described as what?

    a. the positive pole in the Coolidge tube

    b. a lead disk that limits the size of the x-ray beam

    c. is used to screen out long wavelengths

    d. an open-ended extension that is attached to the x-ray tubehead

55. Taking one radiograph on an emergency patient who is pregnant is acceptable if what precautions are followed?

    a. the patient has a digital radiograph taken

    b. the patient is properly draped with a lead apron

    c. the patient has a clearance from her obstetrician

    d. none of the above; the pregnant patient is never to have radiographs

56. An atom can be best described as what?

    a. a simple substance that contains an atomic number

    b. the smallest particle of an element that can retain the properties of that element

    c. positively charged and neutral particles

    d. negatively charged subatomic particles

57. Primary radiation is emitted from what item?

    a. x-ray tubehead

    b. control panel

    c. aluminum filter

    d. film packet

58. The following biological damage may occur when a patient is exposed to radiation.

    a. cell death

    b. mutation of cells

    c. carcinogenesis or cancer causing cells

    d. any of the above

59. When exposing radiographs for a pediatric patient, the exposure time is usually adjusted in what way?

    a. It is increased.

    b. It is decreased.

c. It stays the same.

d. The kilovoltage is set higher.

60. Part of the safety protocol that is set for the protection of patients in the exposure of radiographs might be what?

    a. educational standards set for personnel who perform radiographic procedures

    b. regular inspecting of radiographic equipment

    c. adhering to the ALARA standard

    d. All of the above are safety protocols for the benefit of the patient.

61. A roentgen is considered to be what when talking about dental radiograph?

    a. a special unit of exposure to radiation measured in air

    b. a traditional unit of measurement

    c. equal to one rad times the unit of absorbed dose

    d. equal to six coulombs of radiation

62. When the lead apron is not in use, how should it be stored?

    a. folded neatly and stored on a shelf

    b. in the darkroom

    c. hung on a wire-type hanger

    d. draped over a sturdy rod

63. A lead collimator performs which of the following functions?

    a. It restricts the spread of the x-ray beam to no more than 2.75 inches.

    b. It filters out secondary radiation.

    c. It directs the primary beam toward the patient.

    d. It filters out low-level waves.

64. Which term describes the process by which unstable atoms undergo decay in an effort to obtain nuclear stability?

    a. radioactivity

    b. radiolucent

    c. ionization

    d. absorption

65. Who is the only person allowed to hold the film sensor during exposure?

    a. the dentist

    b. the patient

    c. the dental assistant

    d. the receptionist

66. In normal dental radiographic procedures, the principal hazard to the operator is produced by which type of radiation?

    a. direct radiation

    b. scattered radiation

    c. gamma radiation

    d. alpha radiation

67. Which of the following is designed to restrict the size of the x-ray beam?

    a. a dosimeter

    b. a filter

    c. a collimator

    d. a primary beam restrictor

68. What kind of material is the collimator made out of?

    a. copper

    b. tungsten

    c. samarium

    d. lead

Section III:
Radiation Safety for Patients and Operators – Answers and Rationales

1. Who has the legal responsibility for all acts and services performed in the dental office?

   d. **The dentist is ultimately responsible for any and all acts and services that are performed by any of her or his employees.**

2. Which of these terms best describes the x-rays that are coming directly from the focal spot on the target of the x-ray tube?

   c. **primary beam – X-rays originate from the focal spot.**

3. Who is the only person who should be in the path of the primary beam?

   b. **The patient should be the only person in the path of the primary beam. The operator should stand at least 6 feet away from the primary beam and out of the path.**

4. What is the device that restricts the size of the x-ray beam called?

   CB. **The aluminum in the filter absorbs the low energy, long wavelength x-rays (photons) and allow the high energy, short wavelength x-rays (photons) to pass through the filter.**

5. What material is the collimator made of?

   d. **lead – The collimator is made of lead and restricts the useful beam.**

6. The purpose of the collimator is to

   a. **shape the x-ray beam and restrict its size as it is emitted.**

7. The purpose of the filter is to

   b. **remove many of the long-wavelength x-rays that are not useful during exposure.**

8. Which of these is not an event that follows major exposure to radiation?

   a. **A dose-response period is a useful way to plot the dosage administered with the response of damage produced in order to establish acceptable levels of exposure.**

9. Which of these is the earliest detectable symptom of excessive radiation exposure?

   a. **Erythema or redness in the immediate area of exposure is the earliest detectable symptom of excessive radiation exposure.**

10. Which of these is not considered to be a possible long-term effect of exposure to radiation?

    b. **Arthritis has not been linked to long-term effects of exposure to radiation.**

11. Radiation injuries that do not appear in the person irradiated but occur in future generations are called

    c. **Genetic effects refers to the genetic outcome passed on to future generations.**

12. The earliest detectable physical change due to a large radiation exposure is

    d. **A drop in lymphocyte count would be an indication of the earliest detection of radiation exposure because rapidly dividing cells are the most prone to damage.**

13. Those effects that appear within a matter of minutes, days, or weeks are called

    a. **Acute effects are effects that have a rapid onset. The other three choices all refer to effects that are seen later on.**

14. The cylindrical cone that indicates the direction of the central beam of radiation is also called the

    a. **The PID, also called the position indicating device, is the long, tubular device that is attached to the end of the tubehead where the primary beam is emitted.**

15. Another form of radiation which is given off by any matter irradiated with x-rays is

    b. **Secondary or scatter radiation is the radiation that is emitted from any item that has been exposed to radiation.**

16. Kilovoltage is best described as

    a. **the measurement of electromotive force, equal to 1000 volts. – The kVp setting is one of the most important factors that determines the image contrast, as well as dosage to the patient.**

17. When a cell is damaged by radiation,

    b. **it may repair the damage and operate normally. – In some instances, a cell can repair itself after damage by radiation.**

18. If radiation causes damage to a cell and the cell is not effectively repaired,

    c. **the cell may be removed by the immune system. –Damaged cells are oftentimes removed naturally by the body.**

19. The mechanism that cases damage to cells from radiation exposure is

    a. **ionization – Ionization is the high-energy radiation capable of producing ionization in substances through which it passes.**

20. Genetic effects of radiation appear in the future generation of the exposed person as a result of radiation damage to the

   a. reproductive cells.

21. Name the biggest cause of unnecessary radiation over-exposure.

   c. taking radiographs just because "the patient is due"

22. The maximum permissible dose of radiation per year for dental healthcare workers should not exceed

   a. 5 rems per year.

23. To maximize operator safety during patient exposure, the operator should

   b. stand at least 6 feet away from the patient's head.

24. Which of the following is not a personal monitoring device:

   c. PID device – The PID is the position indicating device, which is the tube that extends from the tubehead of the x-ray machine. This is aimed at the patient during radiographic exposure.

25. The three major elements that make up the x-ray machine are

   b. the vacuum tube, the high-voltage power source, and the operating console.

26. An atom is defined as

   a. the fundamental unit of any element; composed of the nucleus and orbiting electrons.

27. Ionization occurs when

   d. an electrically neutral atom loses an electron and becomes a positively charged ion and the free electron a negative ion, at which time it can interact with live tissue.

28. The operating console

   a. is the control unit, which works to manage the currents, voltage, and timer.

29. Due to the energy within them, x-rays use which type of waves to break through the many layers of body tissues?

   b. Electromagnetic waves, in relation to x-rays, carry with them higher-frequency and shorter wavelengths and have greater penetrating ability than radiation with lower energy.

30. Which of the following is not a source of radiation exposure?

   d. Ultrasonic instrument cleaner does not emit radiation; it emits ultrasonic waves.

31. A film badge is

   a. worn by the operator and is turned in to a monitoring company that will test the badge for exposure.

32. What is the purpose of a personal monitoring device?

   d. It monitors how much radiation an individual operator is being exposed to in a given timeframe. – The monitoring device is sent out at regular intervals for evaluation by an outside source.

33. The ALARA principle, as it relates to operator safety, is followed by

   d. all of the above – All of the above are observed when following the ALARA principle as it relates to operator safety.

34. Ionizing radiation has the potential to produce biological damage

   d. A and B only – X-rays can detach from their larger parts, which creates an imbalance in a normally stable cell.

35. Which term best describes radiation of natural origin?

   a. background radiation – Background radiation is everywhere. It is emitted from such sources as the sun, computer monitors, television screens, and some electronic appliances.

36. Which of these cells is most radiosensitive?

   c. red blood cells – Out of all the cells listed, these are the most sensitive to radiation. Due to their actively dividing status, they can be more sensitive to destruction.

37. Which of these cells is most radioresistant?

   b. muscle cells – Out of the cells listed, these are the most radioresistant. They are least affected to radiation exposure.

38. Which of the tissues that can be in the path of the dental x-ray beam is most radioresistant?

   d. the enamel of the teeth – The enamel of the teeth is radioresistant due to its lack of dividing cells. Enamel is a hardened, calcified matrix and does not contain rapidly dividing cells.

39. The tissue that is most sensitive to radiation is

   c. bone – Due to the high red blood cell formation, bone tissue can be very radiosensitive.

40. Which of these factors has no effect on determining the extent of radiation injury?

   c. the type of film used – The type of film used has no bearing on the extent to which radiation injury can occur.

41. Direct effects of radiation

   a. include damaging effects on a biological, cellular, or molecular level.

42. The letters ALARA stand for

   c. as low as reasonably achievable – All dental offices and those using radiography equipment must adopt the philosophy of ALARA, which is an acronym for "as low as reasonably

achievable." This means that the lowest dosage of radiation exposure to the patient and operator while achieving a diagnostic radiograph is the main objective.

43. What would be a common way to monitor the amount of scatter radiation a healthcare worker may be exposed to?

   a. dosimeter badge

44. Where is the safest position for an operator while exposing an intraoral film?

   d. at a 45-degree angle on the opposite side of the patient

45. The physical effect of radiation is

   a. cumulative.

46. Which of the following group of tissues can be considered the MOST sensitive to radiation exposure?

   d. lymphoid, reproductive cells, and bone marrow

47. For radiation exposure, kilovotage (kV) can be best described as

   b. It determines the quality of penetrating power of the central beam.

48. The ALARA concept emphasizes using the _____ amount of radiation exposure possible.

   a. lowest

49. What is the lead disk that is placed over the opening of the x-ray head referred to?

   C. lead collimator

50. Which item is used to absorb low-energy x-rays that have little penetrating power?

   B. aluminum filter

51. The best way to protect the patient from radiation exposure to the reproductive and thyroid areas is to ensure what happens?

   D. Use a lead apron with thyroid collar attached.

52. To increase the penetrating quality of an x-ray beam, the auxiliary must do which of the following?

   a. increase kVp (kilovoltage peak)

53. Scatter radiation is what type of radiation?

   a. secondary radiation

54. The position indicating device (PID) can be best described as what?

   d. an open-ended extension that is attached to the x-ray tubehead

55. Taking one radiograph on an emergency patient who is pregnant is acceptable if what precautions are followed?

   b. the patient is properly draped with a lead apron – It is safe to take a needed radiograph to diagnose a dental condition if the patient is properly draped and the ALARA principle is followed.

56. An atom can be best described as what?

   b. the smallest particle of an element that can retain the properties of that element

57. Primary radiation is emitted from what item?

   a. x-ray tubehead

58. The following biological damage may occur when a patient is exposed to radiation.

   d. any of the above – Cell death, mutation of cells, and some forms of cancer can all be considered biological damage that may occur during radiation exposure.

59. When exposing radiographs for a pediatric patient, the exposure time is usually adjusted in what way?

   b. It is decreased because bone density and tissue thickness are less on a pediatric patient than on an adult patient.

60. Part of the safety protocol that is set for the protection of patients in the exposure of radiographs might be what?

   d. All of the above are safety protocols for the benefit of the patient.

61. A roentgen is considered to be what when talking about dental radiograph?

   a. a special unit of exposure to radiation measured in air

62. When the lead apron is not in use, how should it be stored?

   d. draped over a sturdy rod – The lead apron should never be folded or rolled up.

63. A lead collimator performs which of the following functions?

   a. It restricts the spread of the x-ray beam to no more than 2.75 inches.

64. Which term describes the process by which unstable atoms undergo decay in an effort to obtain nuclear stability?

   a. radioactivity

65. Who is the only person who should hold the film sensor during exposure? ?

   b. the patient

66. In normal dental radiographic procedures, the principal hazard to the operator is produced by which type of radiation?

   b. scattered radiation

67. Which of the following is designed to restrict the size of the x-ray beam?

   c. a collimator

68. What kind of material is the collimator made out of?

   d. lead

Section IV: Infection Control

This section of the Radiation Health and Safety component of the Certified Dental Assisting Examination consists of 22% or 22 of the 100 multiple-choice items. The questions related to this section of the examination are based upon your knowledge of the following:

- Standard precautions for equipment
- Standard precautions for patients and operators

Quick Review Outline

A. Standard precautions for equipment
   1. The dental assistant should be able to select infection-control techniques and barriers to minimize cross-contamination in the operatory according to ADA/CDC and OSHA guidelines.
      a. The Centers for Disease Control and Prevention (CDC) has published infection-control guidelines. These guidelines recommend that you treat everyone as if known to be infectious. The CDC's infection-control guidelines that directly relate to dental radiology include:
         i. using protective barriers
         ii. wearing protective attire
         iii. frequent hand washing
         iv. sterilization and disinfection of instruments
         v. cleaning and disinfecting dental units and the operatory environmental surfaces
   2. Demonstrate an understanding of barriers used to minimize cross-contamination during radiographic procedures according to ADA, CDC, and OSHA guidelines for conventional and digital radiography.
B. Standard precautions for patients and operators
   1. Demonstrate an understanding of infection control for radiographic procedures according to ADA, CDC, and OSHA guidelines for conventional and digital radiography.
      a. Other sources of x-radiation the operators and other staff may be exposed to while working may include:
         i. computer screens
         ii. television screens
         iii. microwaves
   2. Describe infection-control techniques used during radiographic exposure and processing following ADA, CDC, and OSHA guidelines such as:
      a. barriers on all surfaces that cannot be disinfected or sterilized.
      b. sterilize all film-holding devices.
      c. disposal of single-use items.
      d. using overgloves or clean hands when handling the patient's chart.
      e. washing hands before and after donning gloves.
      f. using gloves, goggles, mask, gown, and protective eyewear during patient contact and in the darkroom.
      g. use an approved sterilant or disinfectant with nitrile gloves during decontamination procedures.

Important Objectives to Know

- Understand the practice of infection control for radiographic processing and following ADA/CDC and OSHA guidelines.
- Be familiar with the maintenance and infection control of digital radiography equipment.

Study Checklist

1. Review your textbook chapter on radiology.
2. Review OSHA guidelines as they refer to infection-control procedures during exposure and processing of radiographs.
3. Review ADA and CDC guidelines as they relate to infection control during exposure and processing of radiographs.

Section IV: Infection Control – Review Questions

Use the Answer Sheet found in Appendix A.

1. Gloves should be worn when exposing dental radiographs to prevent skin contact with
   a. blood.
   b. saliva.
   c. mucous membranes.
   d. all of the above.

2. Which of these terms describes efforts made to reduce disease-producing microorganisms to an acceptable level?
   a. sterilization
   b. asepsis
   c. disinfection
   d. sepsis

3. The best method for sterilizing instruments that come into contact with saliva or blood is by
   a. autoclaving.
   b. wiping with alcohol.
   c. washing with soap and water.
   d. immersing in an ADA-approved surface disinfectant.

4. Which of these items is not suitable for sterilization?
   a. film packet
   b. Rinn film holders
   c. hemostat
   d. mouth mirror

5. Sterilization of radiographic film holding equipment kills pathogens found in the following fluids.
   a. blood
   b. saliva
   c. purulent exudate
   d. any of the above body fluids

6. Digital x-ray sensors
   a. cannot be sterilized.
   b. are sealed and waterproofed.
   c. must be covered with a barrier.
   d. all of the above.

7. 7. Which of the following describes the potential for cross-contamination in dental radiology?
   a. high
   b. low
   c. not a concern in a typical dental setting
   d. cannot be reduced

8. According to the ADA guidelines, how should each patient be treated?
   a. as not being a source of infection
   b. as infectious based on suspicious medical history
   c. as potentially infectious
   d. as a source of noncommunicable disease

9. In infection control, how are radiograph heads or PIDs categorized?
   a. critical
   b. semicritical
   c. noncritical
   d. hypercritical

10. According to the current CDC guidelines, gloves should be worn when taking radiographs
    a. only if the patient has a communicable disease.
    b. only if you are using a digital x-ray sensor.
    c. always, no matter the situation.
    d. never indicated.

11. How should film-holding and positioning devices be treated before patient use?
    a. heat sterilization if possible
    b. disinfection with low-level disinfectant
    c. disinfection with medium-level disinfectant
    d. simple cleaning with antimicrobial soap and water

12. What are the minimum infection-control measures recommended for digital radiology sensors?
    a. FDA-cleared barriers only between patients
    b. heat sterilize and high-level disinfect between patients
    c. clean only between patients
    d. FDA-cleared barriers and clean and disinfect with EPA-registered hospital intermediate-level disinfectant between patients

13. How should contaminated surfaces be cleaned and disinfected?
    a. with soapy water
    b. with alcohol-based wipes
    c. with low- to intermediate-level disinfectant
    d. with hydrogen peroxide

14. With which of the following do standard precautions apply when taking dental radiographs?
    a. only patient with bleeding
    b. all patients
    c. Radiography does not require standard precautions.
    d. only symptomatic patients

15. Which of the following is true of infection-control practices in dental radiology?
    a. They are identical to those used in the dental operatory.
    b. They require sterile technique.
    c. They are not necessary if surgery is not contemplated.
    d. They are not required for minimal contact with blood.

16. To which of the following do standard precautions NOT apply?
    a. body fluids
    b. secretions
    c. sweat
    d. mucous membranes

17. Glove powder can affect the emulsion layer of dental radiographs, causing which event?
    a. fogging
    b. fading
    c. artifacts
    d. radiolucency

18. Which of the following is an advantage of surface barriers in infection control?
    a. reduces the need for universal precautions
    b. shortened patient turnaround time
    c. use of lower-level disinfectants
    d. requires lower-level certification

19. Which of the following is a potential source of cross-contamination when preparing for dental radiographs?
    a. unit dose supplies
    b. control panels on radiology equipment
    c. surface barriers
    d. disposable film holders

20. Which of the following equipment can be protected with surface barriers?
    a. intraoral camera
    b. x-ray cone
    c. bite tabs
    d. automatic processor

21. How should exposed films be transported?
    a. in a disposable container
    b. in a reusable container
    c. by gloved hands
    d. by a dental assistant only

Section IV: Infection Control – Answers and Rationales

1. Gloves should be worn when exposing dental radiographs to prevent skin contact with

   d. all of the above – Gloves should always be worn during radiographic procedures to prevent contact with blood, saliva, and mucous membranes.

2. Which of these terms describes efforts made to reduce disease-producing microorganisms to an acceptable level?

   c. disinfection – This does not completely eliminate disease-producing organisms like sterilization would accomplish but rather brings the bacteria load down to an acceptable level.

3. The best method for sterilizing instruments that come into contact with saliva or blood is by

   a. autoclaving – Autoclaving, when executed properly, will completely render an item pathogen free. Alcohol, soap and water, and disinfectant only leave instruments sanitized or disinfected, not free from pathogenic organisms.

4. Which of these items is not suitable for sterilization?

   a. film packet

5. Gloves should be worn when exposing dental radiographs to prevent skin contact with which body fluid?

   d. any of the above body fluids

6. Digital x-ray sensors

   d. all of the above.

7. Which of the following describes the potential for cross-contamination in dental radiology?

   a. high – The potential for cross-contamination is always considered high.

8. According to the ADA guidelines, how should each patient be treated?

   c. as potentially infectious – All patients are considered infectious.

9. In infection control, how are radiograph heads or PIDs categorized?

   c. noncritical – They do not come into direct contact with the patient's oral cavity.

10. According to the current CDC guidelines, gloves should be worn when taking radiographs

    c. always, no matter the situation.

11. How should film-holding and positioning devices be treated before patient use?

    a. heat sterilization if possible – Since they come into contact with patient body fluids, they must be heat sterilized if possible.

12. What are the minimum infection-control measures recommended for digital radiology sensors?

    d. FDA-cleared barriers and clean and disinfect with EPA-registered hospital intermediate level disinfectant between patients.

13. How should contaminated surfaces be cleaned and disinfected?

    c. with low- to intermediate-level disinfectant

14. With which of the following do standard precautions apply when taking dental radiographs?

    b. All patients should be considered infectious.

15. Which of the following is true of infection-control practices in dental radiology?

    a. They are identical to those used in the dental operatory.

16. To which of the following do standard precautions NOT apply?

    c. sweat

17. Glove powder can affect the emulsion layer of dental radiographs, causing which event?

    c. artifacts

18. Which of the following is an advantage of surface barriers in infection control?

    c. use of lower-level disinfectants

19. Which of the following is a potential source of cross contamination when preparing for dental radiographs?

    b. control panels on radiology equipment

20. Which of the following equipment can be protected with surface barriers?

    a. intraoral camera

21. How should exposed films be transported?

    a. in a disposable container

CHAPTER 3 — INFECTION CONTROL

The Infection Control component of the Certified Dental Assisting Examination consists of 100 multiple-choice items. There are three content areas of focus in this component of the DANB examination. These content areas are:

- Patient and Dental Health Care Worker Education (10% or 10 questions)
  - Demonstrate understanding of infectious disease and their relationship to patient safety and occupational risk.
  - Demonstrate understanding of the procedures and services being delivered and their consequences to the patient, family, other patients, and oral health care personnel.
  - Demonstrate understanding of the need for immunization against infectious diseases.

- Standard/Universal Precautions and the Prevention of Disease Transmission (60% or 60 questions)
  - Prevent cross-contamination and disease transmission (20% or 20 questions)
  - Maintaining aseptic conditions (10% or 10 questions)
  - Demonstrate an understanding of instrument processing (15% or 15 questions)
  - Demonstrate an understanding of asepsis procedures (15% or 15 questions)

- Occupational Safety (30% or 30 questions)
  - Follow the standards and guidelines of occupational safety for dental office personnel.
  - Incorporate all safety measure when using chemical and physical hazards.
  - Maintain and document a quality-assurance (quality-improvement) program for infection control and safety throughout the dental office.

This chapter reviews universal precautions and protective barriers, minimum standards for infection control in dentistry, hazard communication, and general office safety. Sterilization and housekeeping procedures, along with biological monitoring, are also discussed. It is anticipated that this component of the examination will take 1.25 hours to complete. This chapter provides an outline and review of the testing topics and objectives on the Infection Control component of the DANB exam.

Section I: Patient and Dental Health Care Worker Education

This section of the Infection Control portion of the Certified Dental Assisting Examination consists of 10% or 10 of the 100 multiple-choice items. The questions related to this section of the infection control examination are based upon your knowledge of the following.

- Demonstrate an understanding of infectious diseases and their relationship to patient safety and occupational risk.
- Demonstrate an understanding of the procedures and services being delivered and their consequences to the patient, family, other patients, and dental health care personnel.
- Demonstrate an understanding of the need for immunization against infectious diseases such as hepatitis A, B, C, D, E, HIV/AIDS, and other diseases you may encounter in the dental field.

Key Terms

communicable disease – a disease that is infectious and can be transmitted from person to person

cross-contamination – spread of an infection from a person or object to another person

direct contact – touching or firsthand contact with a potentially infectious microorganism

hepatitis – inflammation of the liver that is caused by several viruses

herpes – an infectious viral disease

human immunodeficiency virus (HIV) – a virus that destroys cells of the immune system

immunization – a process that increases an individual's resistance to a particular disease

infection control – methods to eliminate or reduce the transmission of infectious microorganisms

personal protective equipment (PPE) – items that should be worn to protect against contact with all body fluids

Quick Review Outline

A. Infectious diseases and their relationship to patient safety, the dental health care team, and preventing occupational risks

1. The dental assistant should have a thorough knowledge of all infectious diseases that are commonly encountered in the dental office. Protecting all team members and the patient is of great concern. Disease can easily be spread in different ways, and it is the responsibility of the dental assistant to be aware of the disease, its mode of transmission, and precautions to minimize an exposure.

   a. Hepatitis A – inflammation of the liver caused by the hepatitis A virus (HAV). HAV is usually transmitted from person to person by food or drink that has been contaminated with the feces of a person with hepatitis A. This type of transmission is called the "fecal-oral route." The virus is more easily spread in areas where there are poor sanitary conditions or where adequate personal hygiene is not observed. Consuming food or water infected by the virus, using IV drugs, and participating in sexual practices that involve oral/anal contact can all be modes of direct contact with the virus. If you have been exposed to the hepatitis A virus, symptoms will usually show up in 2 to 6 weeks after exposure. They are mild and can last for several months. A physician can initiate a series of tests to confirm infection. Then rest and a diet eliminating alcohol, acetaminophen, and high-fat foods is recommended. Most people will recover within 3 months, with nearly all patients fully recovered within 6 months. There is no cure for hepatitis A, but there is full recovery. When treating patients, always use personal protective equipment such as goggles, gloves, gown, and a mask.

   b. Hepatitis B – like hepatitis A, hepatitis B affects the liver and is spread through blood, semen, vaginal secretions, saliva, and other body fluids of someone who already has a hepatitis B infection. In the dental field, this is the most common type of hepatitis that is spread during dental procedures. Symptoms can range from no symptoms to severe illness. For those who have no symptoms, the virus can easily be spread unknowingly to others; these people are known as chronic carriers of the virus. A physician can run a series of tests to confirm the presence of the hepatitis B virus. There is no treatment once someone has the virus, but there are vaccinations available to protect you before you become exposed. A small percentage of the population cannot recover from the virus and will always carry the virus; these individuals have chronic hepatitis B. Most people can make a complete recovery with no permanent damage to the liver. These individuals have experienced acute hepatitis B. With proper antiviral medications, fluids, and bed rest, these individuals can clear the virus and make a complete recovery. When treating patients, always use personal protective equipment such as goggles, gloves, gown, and a mask.

   c. Hepatitis C – also a blood-borne disease that damages the liver; rarely seen in the dental field. Patients who have hepatitis C suffer from the same symptoms as those who have hepatitis B. Treatment includes medications of the antiviral variety. These medications can create a number of side effects and may manifest themselves in the mouth and create additional challenges to the dental care you are providing. Examine a patient's health history closely and always observe universal precautions and follow the blood-borne pathogens standard. When treating patients, always use personal protective equipment such as goggles, gloves, gown, and a mask.

d. Hepatitis D – Hepatitis D is a form of liver inflammation that occurs only in patients who also are infected by the hepatitis B virus. Infection by the hepatitis delta virus (HDV) either occurs at the same time as hepatitis B develops or develops later when infection by hepatitis B virus (HBV) has entered the chronic (long-lasting) stage. When treating patients, always use personal protective equipment such as goggles, gloves, gown, and a mask (Table 3-1).

Table 3-1: Types of Viral Hepatitis

Disease & Cause	Transmission	Symptoms	Prevention	Long-Term Effects
Viral Hepatitis A (HAV)	Human feces of persons with HAV being transmitted to oral cavity of other person. Example: not washing hands after using bathroom and then preparing food.	Fatigue, loss of appetite, fever, nausea, diarrhea, and jaundice.	• Hepatitis A vaccine recommended for people 12 months and older. • Wash hands. • Immune globulin can be taken within 2 weeks of contact.	• No chronic infection. • Have it only once.
Viral Hepatitis B (HBV)	• Blood from infected person enters a person who is not infected. • Spread through contaminated needles, or other sharps • Sex. • Infected mother to baby during birth.	Fatigue, loss of appetite, fever, nausea, vomiting, joint and abdominal pain, and jaundice. Approximately 1/3 of infected persons have no symptoms.	• Hepatitis B vaccine. • Use of latex condom during sexual activity. • Don't shoot drugs and share needles. • Don't share items that may have blood on them.	• 15–25% will die from chronic liver disease. • High rate of chronic liver disease in infants born to infected mothers.
Viral Hepatitis C (HCB)	• Blood from infected person enters a person who is not infected. • Spread through contaminated needles, or other sharps. • From infected mother to baby during birth. • It can be spread through sexual activity but that is rare.	Fatigue, loss of appetite, nausea, abdominal pain, dark urine, and jaundice.	• No vaccine • Don't shoot drugs and share needles. • Don't share items that may have blood on them. • Wash hands.	• Chronic infection in 55–85% of infected individuals. • 1–5% may die. • Leading indication for liver transplant. • Leading indication for liver transplant. • Uncommon in the United States.
Viral Hepatitis D (HDV)	Same as viral hepatitis B: • Blood from infected person enters a person who is not infected. • Spread through contaminated needles, or other sharps. • Sex. • Infected mother to baby during birth.	Fatigue, loss of appetite, nausea, vomiting, joint and abdominal pain, jaundice and dark urine.	• Hepatitis B vaccine. • Education to reduce risk behaviors.	If co-infection with HBV, the individual may have more severe symptoms and is more likely to have chronic liver disease.
Viral Hepatitis E (HEV)	Same as HAV: Human feces of persons with HAV being transmitted to oral cavity of other person. Example: not washing hands after bathroom and then preparing food.	Fatigue, loss of appetite, nausea, vomiting, dark urine, and jaundice.	• No vaccine • Wash hands.	• No long-term infection. • More severe in pregnant women in their third trimester.

This information was taken from the Centers for Disease Control Web site fact sheets for Viral Hepatitis A–E.

e. Hepatitis E – known as epidemic non-A, non-B hepatitis. Like hepatitis A, it is an acute and short-lived illness that can sometimes cause liver failure. HEV, discovered in 1987, is spread by the fecal-oral route. It is constantly present (endemic) in countries where human waste is allowed to get into drinking water or the food supply. Large outbreaks (epidemics) have occurred in Asian and South American countries where there is poor sanitation. In the United States and Canada, no outbreaks have been reported, but persons traveling to an endemic region may return with HEV. When treating patients, always use personal protective equipment such as goggles, gloves, gown and a mask.

f. HIV/AIDS – The **human immunodeficiency virus (HIV)**, which is a blood-borne infection, is similar to other viruses in that it invades healthy host cells and replicates itself. The cells that HIV invades are the T-cells or CD4 cells, which are the cells that your body uses to fight infection. When these cells are depleted, secondary infection occurs and the HIV virus manifests itself into the acquired immune deficiency syndrome – or, as it is better known, as AIDS. There is no cure. The virus is spread much the same way hepatitis B and C are spread. Coming into contact with the blood, semen, saliva, vaginal secretions, or any secondary vehicle such as a dirty instrument or needle infected with the virus can cause exposure. The HIV virus is fragile. It cannot live on a countertop or clothing. It must have a live host to replicate. Patients with HIV are susceptible to illness and exposure much more readily than someone who is not infected with the virus. Their immune system is delicate, and care must be taken when treating them in the dental office. A medical clearance from their physician is mandatory before rendering treatment. When treating an HIV patient, wear your goggles, mask, gloves, and gown. Follow the CDC established universal precautions and OSHA sterilization procedures, and there will be no danger of spreading the virus to you or to other patients. When following all of the precautions, it is completely safe to deliver treatment to the HIV patient. You cannot spread the virus through casual contact such as a hug or handshake. When treating patients, always use personal protective equipment such as goggles, gloves, gown, and a mask.

g. **Herpes** – also called HSV – is categorized into two groups, HSV 1 and HSV 2. HSV 1 is most commonly the cause of cold sores on the mouth, while HSV 2 is the usual cause of genital herpes. They are interchangeable, which simply means that they can be transmitted from genitals to the mouth and vice versa. Wearing personal protective equipment is always recommended when treating any patient. However, often assistants will not wear their masks properly (not completely covering the nose) or goggles during the entire patient treatment time, and the HSV fluids become airborne and the live virus attacks the mucous membranes in its path. It can infect the eyes and cause blindness and can infect the nasal passages and cause painful recurring sores. It is highly recommended that when a patient has a weeping herpetic lesion, you **do not** treat the patient but wait until the lesion has dried or crusted over. The active virus in the weeping lesion is highly contagious and can not only be spread to the operator but can also be spread to the patient's eyes, nose, or other exposed areas. A rare form of the virus can infect the fingers; this is called a herpetic whitlow. The use of treatment gloves protects the dental assistant from contracting this form of the virus. When treating patients, always use personal protective equipment such as goggles, gloves, gown, and a mask.

h. tuberculosis (TB) – TB is not a great concern in the dental field. Patients who have active TB should not seek routine dental care and should only receive emergency care in a hospital setting. While TB is a bacterial infection spread through airborne transmission, there is a potential for exposure, but the likelihood of contracting TB during the delivery of dental treatment is very low. TB is a concern when there are large groups of people and close contact with each other is likely. Places such as prisons, colleges, or hospitals are of great concern. When treating patients, always use personal protective equipment such as goggles, gloves, gown, and a mask.

i. SARS – Severe acute respiratory syndrome (SARS) is a serious form of pneumonia. It is caused by a virus that was first identified in 2003. Infection with the SARS virus causes acute respiratory distress (severe breathing difficulty) and sometimes death. Patients who have pneumonia and/or have been traveling to foreign countries only to return with pneumonia should not be treated in the dental office until their infection clears. When treating patients, always use personal protective equipment such as goggles, gloves, gown, and a mask.

j. tetanus – the spore causing tetanus infection comes from the *clostridium tetani* bacteria. It can be found in spore form (dormant) or in a vegetative cell (active). It is usually found in soil, dust, and animal waste. While it is not commonly contracted in the dental field, it can contaminate an open wound from patient contact, or the patient may present with it following dental surgery or previous dental abscess. When treating patients, always use personal protective equipment such as goggles, gloves, gown, and a mask.

k. common cold – This is the most common and oldest disease known to mankind. It is spread by bacteria, and the aerosolization can be inhaled from an infected person. Recovering from the common cold can be both time consuming and debilitating. You can receive secondary infections such as bronchitis and pneumonia, which can complicate getting well, not to mention the time off from work that is needed to properly recuperate. Do not go to work with a fever or chronic cough or runny nose. It is not only dangerous to those you work with and patients you come into contact with, it is also distracting to have a health care worker sniffling or constantly coughing. When you are ill, it is equally important to wear gloves, mask, goggles, and a gown to protect the patient from exposure.

B. Demonstrate an understanding of the procedures and services being delivered and their consequences of disease transmission to the patient, family, other patients, and dental care personnel.

1. **Cross-contamination** is always a concern in the dental office, and spreading pathogens from patients to dentists, dental assistants, dental hygienists, dental laboratory technicians, and other patients is a concern. The opposite can be true in that pathogens can also travel from dental personnel to the patient and their family members. These routes of microbial transmission are as follows:

   a. **direct contact** – An individual has direct contact with the microorganism while performing dental procedures.

   b. indirect contact – An individual contacts the microorganism through another means, such as a contaminated surface, instrument, supplies, or equipment.

   c. inhalation/aerosol – An individual contacts the microorganism through inhalation. This usually happens when the high-speed handpiece or the ultrasonic scaler is used in a dental procedure.

2. Take an updated medical history. Always obtain a thorough medical history. Review specific questions about medications, current and recurrent illness, oral soft tissue lesions, or other infections. If the patient has an active illness, a medical consultation with their physician may be needed before moving forward with any kind of dental care.

3. It is the dental assistant's primary duty to take on the responsibility of infection-control practices in the dental office. Using the correct barriers, using PPE, treating all patients as if they are infectious, and using proper disinfection, proper hand hygiene, and sterilization methods breaks the cycle of infection and eliminates cross-contamination and drastically decreases the potential for the spread of pathogens from patients to dental personnel or from dental personnel to patients, who then can take that pathogen home to their family members.

4. Minimizing the spread of disease between the dental worker and their family should be incorporated into the office routine.

   a. Remove lab jackets and/or uniforms and leave them in the designated work area.

   b. Shower when you get home before coming into close contact with family members.

   c. Seek immediate testing and treatment within 2 hours of any occupational exposure. Managing an occupational exposure is the responsibility of the employer as required by the Occupational Safety and Health Administration.

   d. Protect yourself from any potential exposure from a patient by using PPE and following the OSHA standards.

   e. Stay home if you are running a fever, and seek medical treatment if you think you may have been exposed to a contagious disease.

5. Some procedures can cause secondary infection to the patient. The dental assistant should be familiar with these scenarios and caution the patient when appropriate. Following any surgical procedure, the dental assistant should remind the patient there is an inherent risk of infection and describe to the patient what to look for postoperatively. Inflammation, redness, tenderness, bleeding, and sometimes a foul odor coming from

the surgical site can indicate a secondary infection. If the dental assistant sees signs of an infection while caring for the patient, call the dentist in immediately to evaluate for further treatment.

   a. periodontal surgery
   b. surgical extractions
   c. aggressive prophylaxis procedures such as root planing and scaling
   d. other invasive procedures such as implant surgery or more extensive forms of oral surgery.

> **NOTE** If the patient is immunocompromised, there is always a higher potential for secondary infection, and both the patient and their physician should be advised prior to any dental treatment. There should be written documentation from the physician about your mutual patient and the procedure that is going to be performed prior to any treatment being rendered.

C. Demonstrate an understanding of the need for immunization against infectious disease in the dental office.

   1. It is imperative that anyone who has direct patient care should be prepared to receive the proper immunizations prior to working in that environment. Immunizations for the dental health care worker include:

      a. tetanus/diphtheria every 10 years
      b. hepatitis B vaccination series (if the dental health care worker has not had the series, the employer must furnish this series within 30 days of hiring free of charge to the employee)
      c. boosters for any childhood immunizations that may be due such as measles, mumps, and rubella
      d. seasonal flu immunizations
      e. Chickenpox (*varicella*) immunization should be administered if there was not an immunization acquired during childhood.

   2. Many parents, for personal or religious reasons, do not believe in giving their children childhood immunizations, and therefore their children can be exposed with no protection, and that exposure can be brought to you and vice versa. If you never had any of the childhood immunizations, you can easily pass the infection on to a patient. Some childhood diseases can be life threatening when contracted as an adult.

   3. If an expectant mother is exposed to measles, there is a very high probability that her unborn baby will be born with severe birth defects, and in extreme cases the expectant mother can miscarry or deliver a stillborn child.

> **NOTE** According to the Centers for Disease Control, an immunization record should be kept for each employee reflecting both documented histories and immunizations administered at the provider site.

Important Objectives to Know

1. Understand infectious diseases and their relationship to patient safety and occupational risk.
2. Understand the procedures and services being delivered and their consequences to the patient, family, other patients, and dental health care personnel.
3. Understand the need for immunizations against infectious diseases.

Study Checklist

1. Review the most recent CDC, OSHA, OSAP, EPA, and FDA guidelines.
2. Review infection-control chapters in your textbook.
3. Review all infection-control terminology.
4. Review OSHA Bloodborne Pathogens Standard

Section I:
Patient and Dental Health Care Worker Education – Review Questions

Use the Answer Sheet found in Appendix A.

1. Personal protective equipment for the dental assistant who may come into direct or indirect contact with a patient's blood or saliva include all of the following EXCEPT
   a. protective eyewear.
   b. puncture-proof secondary containers.
   c. facemask and gloves.
   d. disposable gown.

2. A patient presents with a history of HIV. When treating the patient with HIV, it is imperative that
   a. you refer them to another office.
   b. you get clearance from their medical doctor before moving forward with dental treatment.
   c. you sterilize all instruments twice.
   d. b and c.

3. After any surgical procedure, you must
   a. remind patient there is an inherent risk of infection and describe to the patient what to look for postoperatively.
   b. give all postoperative instructions to the person who brought the patient in for treatment.
   c. make sure the patient signs the treatment consent form after treatment is performed.
   d. ask the patient to update their health history after performing treatment.

4. Hepatitis A can be spread by
   a. eating or drinking food or water contaminated with feces.
   b. an infected needle.
   c. touching inanimate objects contaminated with the virus.
   d. an infected person donating blood.

5. A patient comes into the office and states on her health history that she has never had the measles immunization but states that her children currently are infected with the measles virus. Who should not be treating the patient?
   a. the 40-year-old hygienist who was immunized as a child
   b. the 30-year-old assistant who is 6 weeks pregnant and was immunized as a child
   c. the 48-year-old dentist who was immunized as a child
   d. the 22-year-old receptionist who has not been immunized

6. Wearing goggles would be most useful in which situation?
   a. a patient with an active herpetic lesion
   b. a patient with bronchitis
   c. a patient who has a history of aphthous ulcers
   d. a patient who has an upper respiratory infection

7. Tetanus can be found in
   a. soil, dust, and animal waste.
   b. contaminated blood.
   c. the respiratory tract.
   d. oral cavity.

8. Which of the following is the easiest way to contract hepatitis B virus in the dental office?
   a. direct transmission
   b. indirect transmission
   c. droplet infection
   d. airborne infection

9. HIV can be spread by all modes except for which one?
   a. inhalation
   b. sharing a needle
   c. mother to infant
   d. sexual contact

10. Which of the following is not considered a blood-borne pathogen?
    a. hepatitis A
    b. hepatitis B
    c. hepatitis C
    d. HIV

11. Herpetic whitlow is an infection of the
    a. oral cavity.
    b. eyes.
    c. hands/fingers.
    d. ears.

12. The best way to protect yourself against the hepatitis B infection is
    a. vaccination.
    b. wearing gloves.
    c. following the Bloodborne Pathogens Standard.
    d. protective eyewear.

13. Hepatitis B is a communicable disease that can be transmitted by the following organism:
    a. flagella
    b. virus
    c. spore
    d. bacteria

14. If a patient becomes infected as the result of a contaminated instrument, the form of disease transmission that occurred was by
    a. indirect contact.
    b. direct contact.
    c. airborne contact.
    d. droplet contact.

15. How often should you be vaccinated for tetanus?
    a. every year
    b. every 3 years
    c. every 5 years
    d. every 10 years

16. A patient's medical and dental history should be reviewed
    a. before rendering clinical dental care.
    b. prior to submitting insurance forms.
    c. periodically at the recall visit.
    d. only if a surgical procedure is indicated.

17. The reasoning behind obtaining a seasonal flu vaccine is
    a. decreases missed days of work.
    b. protects patients and coworkers.
    c. increases the likelihood the recipient will not contract the virus.
    d. all of the above.

18. A health history should be
    a. reviewed and documented at each visit.
    b. signed by the DDS.
    c. copied and sent to their physician.
    d. kept for a year.

19. It is now mandatory for a dentist/employer to offer the hepatitis B vaccine within how many days of hiring to a new employee?
    a. 5 days
    b. 10 days
    c. 20 days
    d. 30 days

20. Patient-to-patient cross-contamination can occur when a patient closes his or her lips around which of the following?
    a. air/water syringe
    b. saliva ejector
    c. high-velocity evacuator tip
    d. Rinn x-ray holder

21. Major factors that contribute to a patient's resistance to infection include
    a. medications.
    b. immune status.
    c. allergies.
    d. All of the above may contribute.

22. Serious infectious diseases that are of major concern to dental personnel are
    a. HIV.
    b. tuberculosis.
    c. hepatitis B and C.
    d. Any of the above can be a concern.

23. Ultimately, the responsibility for infection control lies with the
    a. patient.
    b. dentist.
    c. dental hygienist.
    d. dental assistant.

24. Which of the following infectious diseases is of the least concern to the dental assistant?
    a. tuberculosis
    b. herpes
    c. HIV
    d. hepatitis B

25. Use of the high-speed handpiece could spread microorganisms through which mode of transmission?
    a. direct contact
    b. indirect contact
    c. inhalation
    d. vector

Section I:
Patient and Dental Health Care Worker Education
– Answers and Rationales

1. Personal protective equipment for the dental assistant who may come into direct or indirect contact with a patient's blood or saliva include all of the following EXCEPT

    b. puncture-proof secondary containers.

2. A patient presents with a history of HIV, when treating the patient with HIV, it is imperative that

    b. you get a clearance from their medical doctor before moving forward with dental treatment – Patients with HIV are susceptible to illness and exposure much more readily than someone who is not infected with the virus. Their immune system is delicate, and care must be taken when treating them in the dental office. A medical clearance is mandatory.

3. After any surgical procedure, you must

    a. remind patient there is an inherent risk of infection and describe to the patient what to look for postoperatively.

4. Hepatitis A can be spread by

    a. eating or drinking food or water contaminated with feces.

5. A patient comes into the office and states on their health history that they have never had the measles immunization but states that their children currently are infected with the measles virus. Who should not be treating the patient?

    b. the 30-year-old assistant who is 6 weeks pregnant and was immunized as a child – Even though she has been immunized, the measles immunization usually requires a booster at the age of 21, and she is also pregnant. The measles virus can pose a severe risk to the developing fetus.

6. Wearing goggles would be most useful in which situation?

    a. a patient with an active herpetic lesion – Active weeping herpetic lesions pose a risk to the mucous membranes of the eyes. If the virus enters the eyes, it can cause blindness.

7. Tetanus can be found in

    a. soil, dust, and animal waste.

8. Which of the following is the easiest way to contract hepatitis B virus in the dental office?

    a. direct transmission

9. HIV can be spread by all modes except for which one?

    a. inhalation

10. Which of the following is not considered a blood-borne pathogen?

    a. hepatitis A

11. Herpetic whitlow is an infection of the

    c. hands/fingers.

12. The best way to protect yourself against the hepatitis B infection is by

    a. vaccination.

13. Hepatitis B is a communicable disease that can be transmitted by the following organism:

    b. virus

14. If a patient becomes infected as the result of a contaminated instrument, the form of disease transmission that occurred was by

    a. indirect contact – The patient contacts the microorganism through another means, such as a contaminated surface, instrument, supplies, or equipment.

15. How often should you be vaccinated for tetanus?

    d. every 10 years

16. A patient's medical and dental history should be reviewed

    a. before rendering clinical dental care.

17. The reasoning behind obtaining a seasonal flu vaccine is

    d. all of the above.

18. A health history should be

    a. reviewed and documented at each visit – An accurate health history is instrumental in providing the best care for your patient.

19. It is now mandatory for a dentist/employer to offer the hepatitis B vaccine within how many days of hiring to a new employee?

    b. 10 days

20. Patient-to-patient cross-contamination can occur when a patient closes his or her lips around which of the following?

    b. saliva ejector – Through a process called "suck back," the patient can loosen biofilm from the inside of the saliva ejector hosing and into their mouth via the suction that is created when they release their lips from the saliva ejector straw. Patients don't normally put their lips around the HVE or three-way syringe.

21. Major factors that contribute to a patient's resistance to infection include

    d. All of the above may contribute – Medications, immune status, and allergies may all contribute to a patient's resistance to infection.

22. Serious infectious diseases that are of major concern to dental personnel are

   d. Any of the above can be a concern.

23. Ultimately, the responsibility for infection control lies with the

   d. dental assistant.

24. Which of the following infectious diseases is of the least concern to the dental assistant?

   a. tuberculosis – While TB is a bacterial infection spread through airborne transmission, there is a **potential for exposure, but the likelihood of contracting TB during the delivery of dental treatment is very low.**

25. Use of the high-speed handpiece could spread microorganisms through which mode of transmission?

   c. inhalation – An individual is at greater risk of contacting the microorganism through inhalation when the high-speed handpiece or the ultrasonic scaler is used in a dental procedure.

Section II: Standard/Universal Precautions and the Prevention of Disease Transmission

This topic of the Infection Control portion of the Certified Dental Assisting Examination consists of 60% or 60 of the 100 multiple-choice items. The questions related to this section of the infection-control examination are based upon your knowledge of the following.

- Prevention of cross-contamination and disease transmission (20% or 20 questions)
- Maintaining aseptic conditions (10% or 10 questions)
- Demonstration of an understanding of instrument processing (15% or 15 questions)
- Demonstration of an understanding of asepsis procedures (15% or 15 questions)

Key Terms

asepsis – the creation of an environment free of pathogens
barriers – devices used to keep infectious materials off people and objects in the dental office setting
disinfection – destruction of some microorganisms; cleaning and sanitizing
hand hygiene – technique of washing or decontaminating the hands of microorganisms
modes of disease transmission – methods by which an infectious disease can contaminate a host
sharps – any objects used in dental treatments that can pierce the skin
sterilization – process by which all forms of life are completely destroyed in a controlled area

Quick Review Outline

A. The dental assistant should have extensive knowledge in the prevention of cross-contamination and disease transmission.

1. Proper hand hygiene techniques

   a. Hands must always be washed between patients (following removal of gloves), after touching inanimate objects likely to be contaminated by blood or saliva from other patients, and before leaving the operatory. The rationale for hand washing after gloves have been worn is that gloves become perforated, knowingly or unknowingly, during use and allow bacteria to enter beneath the glove material and multiply rapidly. For many routine dental procedures, such as examinations and nonsurgical events, hand washing with plain soap appears to be adequate, since soap and water will remove transient microorganisms acquired directly or indirectly from patient contact. For surgical procedures, an antimicrobial surgical hand scrub should be used, and hands should be thoroughly scrubbed for at least 2 minutes, taking care to clean under fingernails using a nail brush.

   b. When gloves are torn, cut, or punctured, they must be removed immediately, hands thoroughly washed, and regloving accomplished before completion of the dental procedure.

   c. Dental personnel who have open lesions or weeping dermatitis should refrain from all direct patient care and from handling dental patient-care equipment until the condition resolves.

   d. Hands should be thoroughly washed before and after each patient. The use of alcohol-based gels may be used when hands are free from bioburden and disinfection only is the goal.

   e. For infection-control reasons, nails should be kept short; avoid wearing acrylic nails and nail polish. One ring is acceptable, but wearing several rings is not recommended, as rings harbor bacteria and compromise glove integrity.

2. Single-use disposable materials and equipment are preferred. These items can be disposed of after one use, thus reducing the risk of cross-contamination. Most of the barrier covers used and some dental instruments are now single-use disposable items.

   a. By definition, a single-use or disposable device is intended to be used on one patient and then discarded. If it is a true disposable device, it is not intended to be cleaned and/or sterilized for reuse. These items are not typically manufactured to be heat tolerant.

b. Generally, the following items are designed to be used only one time and then discarded:
  i. anesthetic cartridges and syringe needles
  ii. impression trays
  iii. scalpel blades
  iv. cotton rolls, gauze, and cotton-tipped applicators
  v. prophy angles, cups, and brushes
  vi. saliva ejectors, high-volume evacuation tips, and air/water syringe tips
  vii. dental dams and matrix bands

> **NOTE** As of this printing, it is still undecided whether burs should be exclusively single use. Some are sold as single use, while others can be reused. Studies indicate that burs cannot be free of bioburden after attempted cleaning, and complete removal of bioburden is the goal of infection control. Disposable burs are quickly becoming the standard of care.

3. Use of barrier techniques, personal protective equipment, dental dams, and other safety equipment
  a. The dental assistant must be able to demonstrate the proper use of environmental protective barriers. Chair, tray, equipment, and instrument covers should be used when a surface cannot effectively be cleaned and sterilized in between patient uses. Some surfaces cannot be cleaned and disinfected appropriately, and the dental assistant should know and understand the concept of applying these barriers. Some examples are as follows (Figure 3-1):
    i. light handle covers – impervious-backed paper, foil, or plastic
      (1) Impervious-backed paper, aluminum foil, or clear plastic wrap may be used to cover surfaces (e.g., light handles or x-ray unit heads) that may be contaminated by blood or saliva and that are difficult or impossible to disinfect. The coverings should be removed (with gloved hands), discarded, and then replaced (after degloving and washing hands) with clean barriers between patients.
    ii. chair covers – can cover the chair completely or only the portion where the patient's head and upper body come into contact with the chair
    iii. HVE and saliva ejector covers – plastic covers that slip over the disposable tip and cover at least 12 inches of the tubing
    iv. curing light covers – plastic covers that cover the entire handle and tip
    v. x-ray head covers – plastic covers that cover the entire x-ray head
    vi. x-ray deadman switch covers – impervious-backed paper that covers the entire deadman switch

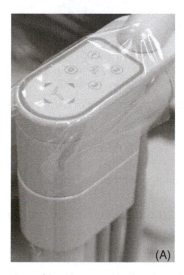
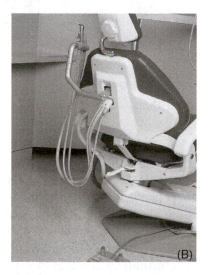

(A) (B)

Figure 3-1 Examples of barrier used in the dental office (A) Barrier covering controls on the dental chair and (B) barriers on the dental unit handpieces

b. Personal protective equipment must be used with all patients to protect the dental assistant from the risk of contamination from bodily fluids.

    i. gloves – When there is a potential for coming into contact with blood, saliva, or mucous membranes, gloves must always be worn. When touching blood-soiled items, body fluids, or secretions, as well as surfaces contaminated with them, you must always wear gloves. Wash your hands before and after donning gloves and change them between patients. Never reuse a pair of gloves.

    ii. Surgical masks and protective eyewear or chin-length plastic face shields must be worn when splashing or spattering of blood or other body fluids is likely to occur.

    iii. Reusable or disposable gowns, laboratory coats, or uniforms must be worn when clothing is likely to be soiled with blood or other body fluids. If reusable gowns are worn, they may be washed using a normal laundry cycle with detergent and bleach. Gowns should be changed at least daily or when visibly soiled with blood, and they should never be worn outside the treatment area.

c. All procedures and manipulations of potentially infective materials should be performed carefully to minimize the formation of droplets, spatters, and aerosols where possible. Use of rubber dams, where appropriate, high-speed evacuation, and proper patient positioning should facilitate this process.

    i. Dental dams or rubber dams are usually made of latex rubber but are also available in non-latex varieties for those patients who are allergic or sensitive to latex. Dental dams are used to isolate the oral cavity during procedures in which moisture (saliva) needs to be controlled. Also, dental dams are effective when chemical agents or small instruments are used in procedures such as in endodontics and the operator wants to discourage the aspiration (inhalation) of these items (Figure 3-2).

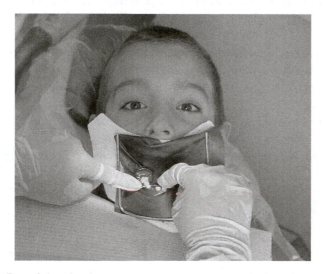

Figure 3-2 Dental dam in place to prevent accidental aspiration of dental materials

B. Maintaining aseptic conditions

1. **Modes of Disease Transmission**

    a. contact transmission – physical transfer of an infectious agent from an infected person to an uninfected person through direct contact or indirect contact

    b. airborne transmission – exposure to an infectious agent through contaminated droplets or dust particles in the air. This can often occur through the use of the dental handpiece.

    c. vehicle transmission – exposure to an infectious agent through inanimate objects such as by contact with a contaminated dental instrument, food, or blood

    d. vector-borne transmission – exposure to an infectious agent by an animate objects such as the bite from a mosquito or a tick (Table 3-2)

Table 3-2: Modes of Transmission

Mode	Examples
Contact	Direct contact of health care provider with patient: • Touching • Secretions from client Indirect contact with fomites: • Clothing • Health care equipment • Instruments used in treatments • Personal belongings • Personal care equipment • Diagnostic equipment
Airborne	Inhaling microorganisms carried by moisture or dust particles in air: • Coughing • Talking • Sneezing • Dental handpiece
Vehicle	Contact with contaminated inanimate objects: • Water • Blood • Drugs • Food • Urine
Vector-borne	Contact with contaminated animate hosts: • Animals • Insects

2. The dental assistant must be able to properly dispose of biohazard and other waste generated in the dental office according to federal regulations.
   a. When handling biopsy specimens, in general, each specimen should be put in a sturdy container and then into a labeled biohazard bag to prevent any leaking during transport. A biohazard label should be affixed to the container and then placed in an impervious bag with a biohazard label placed on the outside. Care should be taken when collecting specimens to avoid contamination of the outside of the container. If the outside of the container is visibly contaminated, it should be cleaned and disinfected.
   b. Disposal of waste materials. All sharps, tissue, bloody gauze, bioburden, or blood should be considered potentially infective and should be handled and disposed of with special precautions. Sharp items (needles, scalpel blades, and other sharp instruments) should be considered potentially infective and must be handled with extraordinary care to prevent unintentional occupational exposures. Disposable syringes and needles, scalpel blades, and other sharp items must be placed in puncture-resistant containers located as close as practical to the area in which they were used. Needles should not be recapped, bent, or broken before disposal (Figure 3-3).

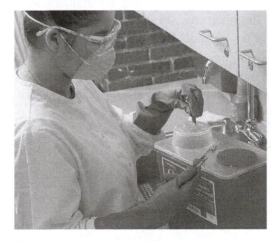

Figure 3-3 All sharps must be placed in a puncture-resistant container

ii. Blood, suctioned fluids, or other liquid waste may be carefully poured into a drain connected to a sanitary sewer system. Other solid waste contaminated with blood or other body fluids should be placed in sealed, sturdy impervious biohazard bags to prevent leakage of the contained items. Such contained solid wastes can then be disposed of according to requirements established by local or state environmental regulatory agencies and published recommendations (Figure 3-4).

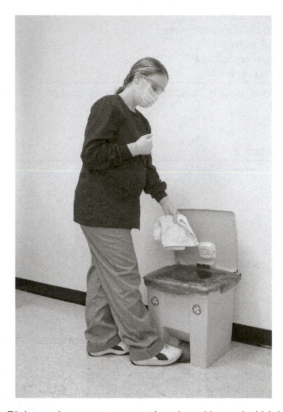

Figure 3-4 Biohazardous wastes must be placed in sealed biohazard bags

    iii. Fixer from film processors is removed by a contract licensed hauler and should never be poured down the sink or disposed of in the trash.

    iv. Amalgam scrap filling materials that contain mercury must be stored under water or mineral in a sealed container and must be either removed by a licensed contract hauler or packaged per guidelines and sent to a designated recycling center.

    v. Managing a mercury spill can best be accomplished by using a mercury spill kit. Mercury should never be placed down a drain or suctioned using the saliva ejector or HVE. Extracted teeth containing amalgam must be disinfected and placed in the amalgam scrap recycling container NOT a biohazard bag. When handling mercury, always wear nitrile gloves, as latex gloves do not provide the protection needed due to the permeability of the latex material.

3. The dental assistant must make sure processed instruments are stored separately from contaminated instruments. There must be a distinct area for "clean" and "dirty" instruments in the sterilization area.

    a. Instruments can be stored in drawers or on trays in a designated "clean" area, which may be in a cabinet, in a drawer, or in the operatory.

    b. Packaged instruments should be dry before they are placed in the storage area. When packages are moist, the instruments may become contaminated either by touching or by laying the package on a contaminated environmental surface.

C. The dental assistant must be proficient and have a solid understanding in performing instrument processing.
 1. Preparation of dental instruments and equipment for sterilization
    a. Wear heavy-duty utility or nitrile gloves.
    b. Discard all single-use items.
    c. Preclean instruments.
    d. Use an ultrasonic cleaner.
    e. Rinse all instruments thoroughly before packaging.
 2. Appropriate methods for sterilization and disinfection of dental instruments, equipment, and supplies
    a. high-level chemical germicides
       i. chemicals registered as sterilant/disinfectant
       ii. have a low surface tension, which means they are able to flow into and penetrate surfaces
       iii. able to penetrate blood and bioburden
       iv. may be used as a holding solution for soiled instruments waiting to be processed
    b. intermediate-level chemical germicides
       i. for surfaces soiled with body fluids
       ii. registered as a "hospital disinfectant"
       iii. labeled as tuberculocidal
       iv. phenols
       v. iodophors
       vi. sodium hypochlorite
    c. low-level chemical germicides
       i. used for general housekeeping
       ii. can be used on floors, countertops, and walls
       iii. disinfection and cleaning dental chairs
       iv. labeled as "hospital disinfectant" but is NOT tuberculocidal (Table 3-3)

Table 3-3: Disinfectant Comparisons

Disinfectant	Level	Advantages	Disadvantages	Time Required for Effectiveness
Chlorine dioxide	High	Rapid disinfection	Corrosive to metals Requires ventilation Irritating to eyes and skin	5–10 minutes
Glutaraldehyde	High	Used to disinfect some impressions Instrument can be submerged Many have a 28-day useful life	Some are corrosive to metal Requires ventilation Irritating to eyes and skin	10–90 minutes
Iodophor	Intermediate	Used as holding solution for impressions	May discolor white or pastel vinyls Surface disinfectant or holding solution Irritating to eyes and skin	10 minutes on surfaces
Sodium hypochlorite	Intermediate	Rapid disinfection	Corrosive to metals Irritating to skin and eyes Diluted solution is unstable, must be mixed daily	5–10 minutes
Phenolics	Intermediate	Available as sprays or liquids	Skin and mucous membrane irritation Cannot be used on plastics	10 minutes
Alcohol	Cleaner only	NA	NA	NA

d. **Sterilization** is the method by which all forms of life are completely destroyed. Any living organism or pathogen is eradicated. "Sterile" is an absolute term. Either an item is sterile or it is not sterile. There are three accepted methods of sterilization in the dental field.

    i. autoclave

        (1) Superheated steam under pressure combined with time for successful autoclaving
            Pressure: 15–20 psi (pounds per square inch)
            Temperature: 250 degrees F
            Time: 20 minutes after the proper pressure and temperature has been reached
            When using sterilization bags (half paper and half plastic), load instruments upright so vapors or steam can penetrate each sterilization pouch evenly. Never stack packages on top of each other or overload the sterilizer.

        (2) Distilled water is used in the autoclave.

        (3) Instruments are dried and wrapped in a sterilization bag or placed in a cassette and wrapped for processing.

        (4) After processing, instruments are removed and allowed to cool and dry.

        (5) Examine door gaskets on a regular basis to ensure that the unit is not leaking or worn out. Keep autoclave supplied with water and clean on a weekly basis (follow manufacturer's recommendation on cleaning and servicing).

    ii. chemclave

        (1) Similar to autoclaving except that chemical vapor is used instead of distilled water
            Pressure: 20–24 psi
            Temperature: 270 degrees F
            Time: 20 minutes

        (2) Instruments must be clean and dry before they are wrapped.

        (3) Instruments can be wrapped in paper/biofilm bags or placed in cassettes.

        (4) A vapor exhaust system is needed to eliminate harmful vapors after decompression of the chemclave.

        (5) Ensure the chemclave is supplied with the designated chemical vapor.

        (6) Follow manufacturer's suggestions on cleaning and maintenance.

    iii. dry heat sterilization

        (1) This method is used when instruments will rust in the autoclave or chemclave.

        (2) Instruments must be clean and dry before they are placed in the dry heat sterilizer.

        (3) Procedure for dry heat sterilization
            160 degrees F for 120 minutes
            170 degrees F for 60 minutes
            Placed in a heat-resistant container
            Timing of the sterilization process begins when the proper temperature is met.

    iv. Cold sterilization is not as common as it once was, but some offices still utilize this form of sterilization for items that cannot tolerate high heat, steam, or chemical vapor. Items such as high-velocity evacuator tips, x-ray rings, Snap-A-Ray holders, and plastic syringes can be safely sterilized using cold sterilant.

        (1) Cold sterilant is usually an FDA-cleared glutaraldehyde or hydrogen peroxide–based solution that is mixed and typically has a 28-day shelf life from the day of activation and/or put into use. For sterilization to be effective, items should be left in the solution for at least 6 hours; no additional items should be added to the solution during this time period.

        (2) Safety precautions should be observed when using all cold sterilant solutions. Gloves, goggles, and chemical-resistant gloves should be worn when using cold sterilant solutions. Follow manufacturer's guidelines when mixing, using, and disposing of all products. Observe the SDS sheet and understand the dangers and first aid associated with these chemicals.

3. Appropriate biological monitoring and process indicators
   a. CDC guidelines regarding proper achievement of sterilization are guaranteed only through biological monitoring. In addition to testing, confirmation from an independent monitoring service is ideal.
   b. Spore testing uses live spores that are harmless but very resistant to heat. Weekly monitoring is recommended. Generally, two strips are used. One strip is run with the instruments and the other is the control strip. Both strips are sent to an outside lab for evaluation. Mechanical failure of sterilization equipment is the number-one reason for incomplete sterilization of dental instruments.
   c. Process indicators are used to identify those instruments that have been processed through the sterilizer. The heat- or vapor-sensitive paper is located on the bags or tape used to seal the bags. There are also individual strips that can be placed inside the sterilization pouch or wrapped cassette that indicate exposure to heat or chemical vapor. This material only indicates whether the instruments were exposed to chemical vapor, steam, or other sterilization chemicals and does not guarantee whether the instruments are sterile (Figure 3-5).

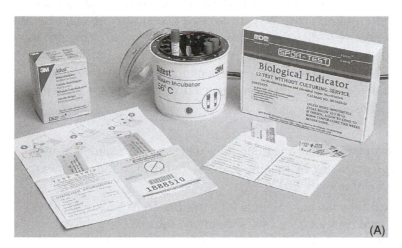
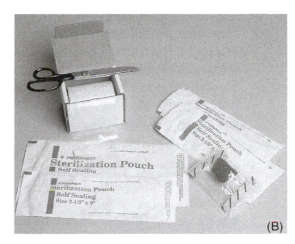

(A)   (B)

Figure 3-5 (A) Biological monitors and (B) process indicators used for dental sterilizers

D. Asepsis Procedures
   1. The dental assistant must be able to prepare surfaces for disinfection by using detergent and disposable toweling to first remove bioburden or visible material from hard surfaces before a high-level disinfectant can be used on the surface. The assistant must then incorporate the spray-wipe-spray method by spraying the surface, wiping the surface, and then spraying again, leaving the surface to air dry.
   2. The dental assistant must be able to understand the use of proper methods for disinfection for environmental surfaces, including the treatment of the dental laboratory, darkroom, and instrument processing and equipment areas. For example, disposable toweling aids in the prevention of spreading contaminants from one surface to the next. High-level disinfectants and cleaners designed to reduce virus and bacterial contaminants should be used when appropriate.
      i. At the completion of work activities, countertops and surfaces that may have become contaminated with blood or saliva should be wiped with absorbent toweling to remove extraneous organic material, then disinfected with a suitable chemical germicide. A solution of sodium hypochlorite (household bleach) prepared fresh daily is an inexpensive and very effective germicide. Concentrations ranging from 5,000 ppm (a 1:10 dilution of household bleach to water) to 500 ppm (a 1:100 dilution) sodium hypochlorite are effective, depending on the amount of organic material (e.g., blood, mucus) present on the surface to be cleaned and disinfected. Caution should be exercised, since sodium hypochlorite is corrosive to metals, especially aluminum. Alternatively, an EPA-approved hospital germicide can also be used to clean hard surfaces. Care should be taken if the germicide contains glutaraldehyde, which is a known carcinogen. Worth mentioning is a word about countertops. Countertops should have designated areas that differentiate between clean (sterilized) and dirty (contaminated) areas.

ii. Routine sterilization of handpieces between patients is desirable; however, not all handpieces can be sterilized. If a handpiece cannot be sterilized, the following procedure can be used. After use, the handpiece should be flushed, then thoroughly scrubbed with detergent and water to remove any bioburden material. It should then be thoroughly wiped with absorbent material saturated with a chemical germicide that is registered with the EPA as a "hospital disinfectant" and is mycobactericidal. The disinfecting solution should remain in contact with the handpiece for a time specified by the disinfectant's manufacturer. Ultrasonic scalers and air/water syringes should be treated in a similar manner between patients. Following disinfection, any chemical residue should be removed by rinsing with sterile water.

iii. laboratories, materials, and impressions – Blood and saliva should be thoroughly and carefully cleaned from laboratory supplies and materials that have been used in the mouth (e.g., impression materials, bite registration), especially before polishing and grinding intraoral devices. Materials, impressions, and intraoral appliances should be cleaned and disinfected before being handled, adjusted, or sent to a dental laboratory. These items should also be cleaned and disinfected when returned from the dental laboratory and before placement in the patient's mouth. Because of the ever-increasing variety of dental materials used intraorally, dental health care workers (DHCWs) are advised to consult with manufacturers as to the stability of specific materials relative to disinfection procedures. A chemical germicide that is registered with the EPA as a "hospital disinfectant" and that has a label claim for mycobactericidal (e.g., tuberculocidal) activity is preferred, because mycobacteria represent one of the most resistant groups of microorganisms; therefore, germicides that are effective against mycobacteria are also effective against other bacterial and viral pathogens.

iv. radiographic darkrooms

2. The dental assistant must understand how to maintain dental water unit lines. Due to accumulation of biofilm within dental water and suction tubing, daily cleaning by running an EPA-approved solution through the lines cuts down on the formation of biofilm within these lines.

i. Because water-retraction valves within the dental units may aspirate infective materials back into the handpiece and water line from the patient's oral cavity, check valves should be installed to reduce the risk of transfer of infective material. While the magnitude of this risk is not known, it is prudent for water-cooled handpieces to be run and to discharge water into a sink or container for 20 to 30 seconds after completing care on each patient. This is intended to physically flush out patient material that may have been aspirated into the handpiece or water line. Additionally, there is some evidence that overnight bacterial accumulation can be significantly reduced by allowing water-cooled handpieces to run and to discharge water into a sink or container for several minutes at the beginning of the clinic day. Sterile saline or sterile water should be used as a coolant/irrigator when performing surgical procedures involving the cutting of soft tissue or bone.

3. The dental assistant must be able to understand the information represented on the Safety Data Sheet that accompanies each chemical agent used in the dental office. A Safety Data Sheet (SDS) is a document that contains information on the potential hazards (health, fire, reactivity, and environmental) and how to work safely with the chemical product. It is an essential starting point for the development of a complete health and safety program. It also contains information on the use, storage, handling, and emergency procedures all related to the hazards of the material. The SDS contains much more information about the material than the label does. SDSs are prepared by the supplier or manufacturer of the material. They are intended to tell what the hazards of the product are, how to use the product safely, what to expect if the recommendations are not followed, what to do if accidents occur, how to recognize symptoms of overexposure, and what to do if such incidents occur. Some examples are as follows:

a. Developer and fixer solutions
b. Cold sterilization solution
c. Chemclave solution
d. Hard-surface disinfectants
e. Ultrasonic solution
f. Suction and waterline cleaning solution

4. The dental assistant must be able to understand what differentiates critical, semicritical, and noncritical items and how they are processed and sterilized.

    a. Critical items cut bone or penetrate soft tissue. This type of instrument carries the highest risk of disease transmission. These instruments should be cleaned and heat-sterilized before each use.

    b. Semicritical items touch only mucous membranes and carry a lower risk of transmission than critical instruments would. They should be cleaned and heat-sterilized before each use. Always use heat-stable semicritical items instead of those items that are heat sensitive when possible. These instruments can be processed using an FDA–cleared sterilant/high-level disinfectants or an FDA–cleared low-temperature sterilization method such as ethylene oxide gas. Single-use instruments are acceptable alternatives.

    c. Noncritical items only contact intact skin. These items have the lowest risk of disease transmission. The dental assistant must make sure that these items are covered with acceptable barriers or cleaned/disinfected after each use with an EPA-registered hospital disinfectant. If bioburden is visible (blood, tissue), an EPA-registered hospital disinfectant with a tuberculocidal claim must be used.

Important Objectives to Know

1. Preventing cross-contamination and disease transmission
2. Proper instrument processing
3. Maintaining aseptic conditions
4. Performing proper sterilization procedures

Study Checklist

1. Review all infection-control terminology.
2. Review and practice procedures related to disinfection, sterilization, instrument processing, hand hygiene, and use of PPE.
3. Review common chemicals and sterilization equipment used in the dental office.
4. Review text chapters for infection control.

Section II: Standard/Universal Precautions and the Prevention of Disease Transmission – Review Questions

Use the Answer Sheet found in Appendix A.

1. Which type of microorganism is highly resistant to heat and chemicals?
   a. viruses
   b. spores
   c. *staphylococci*
   d. yeasts

2. What mode of disease transmission is transmitted through a needle stick?
   a. droplet infection
   b. airborne infection
   c. indirect contact
   d. direct contact

3. The leading cause of sterilization failure in the dental office is
   a. equipment malfunction.
   b. human error.
   c. improper packaging.
   d. oversaturation of chemical during sterilization.

4. Which protective equipment should be worn while cleaning contaminated instruments?
   a. latex gloves and protective clothing
   b. a mask, nitrile utility gloves, protective eyewear, and protective clothing
   c. a mask, protective eyewear, and protective clothing
   d. heavy-duty utility gloves, mask, and eyewear

5. What is the reason for cleaning instruments prior to sterilization?
   a. reduce instrument rust buildup
   b. kill any microorganisms on the working ends of the instruments
   c. increase the chance of complete sterilization of instrument
   d. minimize instrument repair

6. All of the following are true about protective clothing except which one?
   a. It should be worn when coming into contact with blood or other body fluids.
   b. It should be changed after becoming visibly soiled.
   c. It can be taken home each day and cleaned with hot water, soap, and bleach.
   d. It can be worn outside the clinical area.

7. When should surgical gloves be worn?
   a. during any clinical dental office procedure
   b. when there is a potential for contacting blood or body fluids
   c. only when treating a live patient
   d. when assisting with surgical procedures

8. Sterilized instruments should be stored in the following manner:
   a. unwrapped in a designated drawer
   b. loose on a storage tray
   c. in a cassette in the sterilization area
   d. wrapped in a cassette, on a preset tray, or in a drawer

9. A face shield must be worn
   a. for procedures that commonly result in the generation of blood droplets.
   b. during every dental procedure.
   c. only when using the model trimmer or lab engines.
   d. only when cleaning dental instruments.

10. Barriers for light handles and chairs should be
    a. impervious-backed paper or plastic covers.
    b. easy to remove.
    c. adequate coverage for all items that are difficult to clean or disinfect.
    d. all of the above.

11. Sterilization and disinfection of critical instruments
    a. is done only if the doctor requests it.
    b. can be done the next day.
    c. is done after each use.
    d. is only done if the instruments have come into contact with blood.

12. Washing your hands before and after donning gloves increases
    a. the potential for cross-contamination.
    b. the potential for direct contamination.
    c. the potential for the decrease of resident bacteria on hands.
    d. the potential for indirect contamination.

13. Proper spore-testing verification can be accomplished by
    a. reading the vapor indicator on the bag after sterilization is complete.
    b. using a biological monitoring strip and then sending it out for evaluation.
    c. using a heat-indicator tape on the sterilization package.
    d. making sure proper heat and temperature are achieved with the sterilizer.

14. Preventing the spread of disease from the dental office to the general public is best accomplished by
    a. washing your hands regularly.
    b. disinfecting any materials that are sent to the lab.
    c. using personal protective equipment with all patient contact.
    d. all of the above.

15. Suction lines can be cleaned with
    a. a commercial dental evacuation cleaner or bleach-and-water mixture of 1 part bleach to 10 parts water.
    b. ultrasonic cleaner.
    c. cold tap water.
    d. soapy hot water.

16. Sterilization is best defined as
    a. condition of being free from all pathogenic microorganisms.
    b. process by which all forms of life are completely destroyed.
    c. process by which the number of pathogenic organism is reduced to a safe level.
    d. presence of a limited level of pathogenic organisms.

17. Dental units and chairs are generally cleaned
    a. between each and every patient.
    b. at the start of each day.
    c. at the end of each day.
    d. only when visibly soiled.

18. After packaging instruments for sterilization, the autoclave or chemclave should be loaded
    a. slowly to prevent damage to the instrument packs.
    b. by placing instrument packs in an upright position.
    c. with as many instrument packs as possible.
    d. with both wrapped and unwrapped instrument packs.

19. **Asepsis** is defined as the
    a. method for disease transmission.
    b. presence of disease-producing microorganisms.
    c. absence of bacteria, viruses, and other microorganisms.
    d. infection that can spread to other patients.

20. Disposable needles and glass anesthetic cartridges are discarded in a
    a. red biohazard puncture-proof container.
    b. standard garbage can.
    c. red labeled plastic trash bag.
    d. sealable sterilization pouch.

21. Biological monitors for the autoclave should be run
    a. on a daily basis.
    b. on a weekly basis.
    c. on a monthly basis.
    d. not necessary on an autoclave.

22. Personal protective equipment (PPE) may include
    a. gloves, eyewear, and surgical gowns.
    b. oxygen masks.
    c. dental dam.
    d. light-cure sleeve to prevent cross-contamination.

23. Your dentist extracts a tooth that has an amalgam restoration in it. The best way to dispose of the tooth would be to
    a. place it in the biohazard waste.
    b. rinse it off, place it in an autoclave bag, sterilize it, and place it in the trash.
    c. place it into a scrap amalgam container for processing by a recycler.
    d. place it in the sharps container for pick up by a licensed hauler.

24. In the lab, which is the best way to care for the ragwheel?
    a. washing
    b. autoclaving
    c. rinsing and reusing
    d. only A and B together

25. The CDC recommends that you biologically monitor the sterilizer at what interval?
    a. each load
    b. weekly
    c. monthly
    d. yearly

26. Which of the following is not considered acceptable for use as a surface disinfectant in the dental office?
    a. iodophor
    b. chlorine-based products
    c. glutaraldehydes
    d. phenolics

27. A dental anesthetic carpule is considered a sharps item and should be discarded in the sharps container?
    a. only if it is broken.
    b. regardless if its broken or not.
    c. never.
    d. It and never in the regular trash.

28. Which of the following is not true regarding hand washing?
    a. Hands should be washed before and after donning gloves.
    b. Hands should be washed before setting up the barriers for treatment.
    c. Hands do not have to be dried completely before donning gloves.
    d. Hands should be washed in cool water with antimicrobial soap.

29. Nitrile utility gloves are used for
    a. cleaning up spills on countertops and floors.
    b. cleaning instruments that may be contaminated with blood.
    c. housekeeping duties that involve potential contact with blood and tissue.
    d. all of the above.

30. How often should the suction lines be flushed with an EPA-approved solution?
    a. daily
    b. weekly
    c. biweekly
    d. monthly

31. All of the following are disposed of in the sharps container except
    a. used blades.
    b. intact anesthetic carpules.
    c. used needles.
    d. broken medication vials.

32. Using an FDA-approved glutaraldehyde mix, cold sterilization can be achieved by at least
    a. 2 hours of exposure to instruments.
    b. 6 hours of exposure to instruments.
    c. 8 hours of exposure to instruments.
    d. 10 hours or more of total immersion.

33. All of the following reasons are true for using a dental dam except
    a. to isolate one or more teeth for treatment.
    b. to prevent aspiration of endodontic armamentarium.
    c. to maintain patient airway.
    d. moisture control.

34. When using the chemclave, all except the following must be achieved for sterilization to be successful:
    a. recommended time is reached
    b. recommended temperature is reached
    c. recommended pressure is reached
    d. recommended cassettes are used

35. High-level chemical germicides are registered
    a. as sterilants/disinfectants.
    b. disinfectant.
    c. tuberculocidal.
    d. virucidal.

36. Single-use instruments
    a. do not come into contact with intact skin.
    b. are not disposable.
    c. need disinfection at a minimum.
    d. are designed to be used only one time and then discarded.

37. Lab cases such as dentures or partials should be
    a. handled with gloves.
    b. disinfected prior to being placed into the patient's oral cavity.
    c. disinfected before being sent to the lab.
    d. all of the above.

38. When recapping an anesthetic needle, OSHA protocol recommends
    a. using a recapping device.
    b. bending the needle.
    c. using both hands to recap the needle.
    d. allowing the dentist to recap it while you are holding it.

39. Droplet infection can be best described as
    a. occurring with inhalation of aerosol generated during dental procedures.
    b. occurring through a break in the skin.
    c. occurring by touching a contaminated surface.
    d. occurring through a surgical incision.

40. The most common mode of disease transmission that occurs in the dental office is
    a. airborne.
    b. splash or spatter.
    c. direct or indirect.
    d. parenteral.

41. Instruments considered "critical" should always
    a. be disinfected.
    b. be sterilized.
    c. be disposed of according to EPA guidelines.
    d. be placed in the sharps container.

42. Sepsis can be best defined as
    a. the condition of being free from disease-producing microorganisms.
    b. the destruction of all forms of life except those bacterial in nature.
    c. the presence of disease-producing microorganisms.
    d. process by which all forms of life are destroyed.

43. Steam sterilization under pressure can be achieved using a/an
    a. ultrasonic.
    b. autoclave.
    c. chemclave.
    d. ethylene oxide sterilizer.

44. Semicritical instruments
    a. do not penetrate soft tissue.
    b. contact soft oral tissue.
    c. require sterilization or high disinfection after each use.
    d. all of the above.

45. Bloody gauze or tissue must be disposed of by
    a. placing in a sealed Ziploc bag and then the regular trash.
    b. placing in the biohazard waste.
    c. placing in a sharps container.
    d. putting it into the regular trash.

46. The best way to manage a mercury spill is to
    a. suction it up using the HVE.
    b. scoop it into a gloved hand and dispose into the sharps container.
    c. scoop it into a plastic cup and dispose it into a ceramic basin.
    d. use a mercury spill kit.

47. Discarded scrap amalgam is best stored by
    a. throwing it away in the sharps container.
    b. placing it in a plastic bag and then in the operatory garbage.
    c. keeping it in a glass jar with an airtight lid.
    d. storing it under water or fixer in a sealed container.

48. Ultrasonic cleaners are available as
    a. liquids.
    b. enzymatic and nonenzymatic formulations for instrument cleaning.
    c. nonenzymatic effervescing soluble tablets.
    d. all of the above.

49. The preferred method for cleaning hard surfaces would be
    a. saturation of surface and allowed to air dry.
    b. spray and wipe with cloth towel.
    c. disposable toweling and an EPA–registered disinfectant for hard surfaces.
    d. a commercial spray such as Lysol and air dry surface.

50. Mask selection should be based on
    a. the level of protection required.
    b. fit.
    c. breathability.
    d. all of the above.

51. Prior to surgical procedures, **hand hygiene** must be performed with
    a. antimicrobial soap and water with aggressive rubbing.
    b. an alcohol-based hand rub.
    c. plain soap and hot water.
    d. none of the above.

52. In the dental office, the best way to reduce the risk of contracting a communicable disease is to
    a. take a thorough health history.
    b. use disposable items.
    c. wear a face mask, examination gloves, and protective eyewear.
    d. all of the above.

53. The ultrasonic cleaner contains a liquid medium to aid in the removal of debris from instruments. The solution should be changed
    a. at the end of the day.
    b. every other day.
    c. only when it looks dirty.
    d. monthly.

54. Which chemical agent is acceptable for clinical contact surface disinfection?
    a. EPA-registered
    b. OSHA-registered
    c. ISO-registered
    d. ANSI-registered

55. Critical instruments are considered
    a. to contact and penetrate tissues.
    b. to contact mucous membranes and not penetrate tissues.
    c. to contact skin only.
    d. disposable.

56. A curing light emits a visible light, so it is imperative that you wear
    a. a protective face shield.
    b. protective eyeglasses.
    c. protective tinted eyewear.
    d. a mask.

57. Dental handpieces (both high and slow speed) should be sterilized
    a. once a day.
    b. after each patient.
    c. before and after lubrication.
    d. after working on a patient with a communicable disease.

58. Why is it important to dry instrument packages inside the sterilizer after the end of the sterilization cycle?
    a. It prevents microbes from penetrating the moist package.
    b. Prevents instruments from sticking to each other.
    c. Prevents water spots from forming on instruments.
    d. Allows chemical indicators to give a proper reading.

59. When is the most appropriate time to use an alcohol-based hand rub?
    a. only if a sink is available
    b. only if used before using another hand washing agent
    c. only if used after another hand washing agent
    d. only when there is no visible soil on the hands

60. Some patient-care instruments and armamentarium such as blood pressure cuffs, stethoscope, and pulse oximeter are categorized as
    a. critical.
    b. semicritical.
    c. noncritical.
    d. single use.

61. Instruments are sterilized by chemical sterilization for how many minutes at what temperature?
    a. 10 to 20/250
    b. 20 to 30/270
    c. 30 to 60/340
    d. 60 to 120/320

62. Plastic disposable items are designed to be
    a. cold sterilized if constructed of plastic.
    b. never sterilized.
    c. discarded even if placed on instrument tray and not used.
    d. reused if placed on instrument tray and not used for procedure.

63. When using the dry-heat sterilization method, instruments must be dried completely to avoid
    a. cross-contamination.
    b. breakage.
    c. rusting.
    d. dulling of the working end.

64. A steam sterilizer requires which kind of solution?
    a. purified water
    b. EPA-approved solutions
    c. glutaraldehyde
    d. distilled water

65. To "flash autoclave" an instrument, the following must be done:
    a. 8 minutes for a wrapped load at 250 degrees F at 30 psi
    b. 30 minutes for a wrapped load at 250 degrees F at 24 psi
    c. 450 degrees F unwrapped for 12 seconds
    d. 280 degrees F wrapped for 25 minutes

66. Dry-heat sterilization requires how many hours for sterilization?
    a. 2 to 4
    b. 4 to 6
    c. 8 to10
    d. 10 or more

67. Biological indicators used to test steam sterilizers contain
    a. *Bacillus stearothermophilus.*
    b. *Mycobacterium tuberculosis.*
    c. active viruses.
    d. *Streptococcus mutans.*

68. Ethylene oxide is a form of gas sterilization that requires approximately how many hours of exposure to be effective?
    a. 2
    b. 8
    c. 10–16
    d. 24

69. To avoid cross-contamination from patient to patient, it is recommended that you do the following:
    a. Use disposable items when possible.
    b. Clean the dental chair and bracket table between patients.
    c. Use a dental dam when there is a potential for generation of aerosol.
    d. Run the suction lines with an EPA-approved solution at the end of each work day.

70. The fiber-optic light surface on the high-speed handpiece should be cleaned with isopropyl alcohol and a cotton-tip applicator
    a. once a day.
    b. before each use.
    c. after it is sterilized.
    d. after it is cleaned by the ultrasonic.

71. This method of sterilization requires that items must be completely submerged and undisturbed for at least 6 hours for cold sterilization.
    a. ethylene oxide
    b. glass bead sterilizer
    c. steam autoclave
    d. glutaraldehyde

72. When using a chemclave, which liquid product is used during the sterilization process?
    a. deodorized alcohol formaldehyde
    b. distilled water
    c. formalin creosote
    d. anhydrous bleach solution

73. A negative sporicidal test you run on the autoclave comes back as negative. What does this mean?
    a. Sterilization did occur.
    b. Sterilization did not occur.
    c. The control strip was contaminated.
    d. The spore test should be run again.

74. Adequate ventilation is required for which sterilizer?
    a. ethylene oxide
    b. chemclave
    c. dry-heat sterilizer
    d. glass bead sterilizer

75. The type of gloves used during disinfection and cleanup procedures are called
    a. overgloves.
    b. latex gloves.
    c. vinyl gloves.
    d. utility gloves.

Section II: Standard/Universal Precautions and the Prevention of Disease Transmission – Answers and Rationales

1. Which type of microorganism is highly resistant to heat and chemicals?

   b. spores

2. Which mode of disease transmission is transmitted through a needle stick?

   c. indirect contact

3. The leading cause of sterilization failure in the dental office is

   a. equipment malfunction

4. Which protective equipment should be worn while cleaning contaminated instruments?

   b. a mask, nitrile utility gloves, protective eyewear, and protective clothing

5. What is the reason for cleaning instruments prior to sterilization?

   c. increase the chance of complete sterilization of instrument

6. All of the following are true about protective clothing except which one?

   d. It can be worn outside the clinical area.

7. When should surgical gloves be worn?

   b. when there is a potential for contacting blood or body fluids

8. Sterilized instruments should be stored in the following manner:

   d. wrapped in a cassette, on a preset tray, or in a drawer

9. A face shield must be worn

   a. for procedures that commonly result in the generation of blood droplets.

10. Barriers for light handles and chairs should be

    d. all of the above.

11. Sterilization and disinfection of critical instruments

    c. is done after each use.

12. Washing your hands before and after donning gloves increases

    c. the potential for the decrease of resident bacteria on hands.

13. Proper spore-testing verification can be accomplished by

    b. using a biological monitoring strip and then sending it out for evaluation.

14. Preventing the spread of disease from the dental office to the general public is best accomplished by

    a. washing your hands regularly.

15. Suction lines can be cleaned with

    a. a commercial dental evacuation cleaner or bleach-and-water mixture of 1 part bleach to 10 parts water.

16. Sterilization is best defined as

    b. process by which all forms of life are completely destroyed.

17. Dental units and chairs are generally cleaned

    a. between each and every patient.

18. After packaging instruments for sterilization, the autoclave should be loaded

    d. with both wrapped and unwrapped instrument packs.

19. Asepsis is defined as the

    c. absence of bacteria, viruses, and other microorganisms.

20. Disposable needles and glass anesthetic cartridges are discarded in a

    a. red biohazard puncture-proof container.

21. Biological monitors for the autoclave should be run

    b. on a weekly basis.

22. Personal protective equipment (PPE) may include

    a. gloves, eyewear, and surgical gowns.

23. Your dentist extracts a tooth that has an amalgam restoration in it. The best way to dispose of the tooth would be to

    c. place it in a scrap amalgam container for processing by a recycler – Extracted teeth can be placed in the amalgam waste. Never place them in the biohazard, because biohazard waste is usually incinerated, and when amalgam is incinerated, mercury vapors can be released.

24. In the lab, which is the best way to care for the ragwheel?

    d. A and B together: washing and autoclaving – The best way to care for the ragwheel is to clean it thoroughly and then package it and send it through the autoclave after each use. Changing the pumice and cleaning the tub in which the pumice sits needs to be addressed as well.

25. The CDC recommends that you biologically monitor your sterilizer at what intervals?

    b. weekly – Weekly spore testing must be done and sent out for testing by an outside facility. Records of the results should be kept in a binder and stored with other office maintenance records.

26. Which of the following is not considered acceptable for use as a surface disinfectant in the dental office?

    c. glutaraldehydes – This product is designed to be used as a cold sterilizer, with instruments being immersed for at least 6 to 8 hours or more for effectiveness. Used as a surface disinfectant, it can cause nose and eye irritation and may cause breathing difficulties in some people.

27. dental anesthetic carpule is considered a sharps item and should be discarded in the sharps container?

    d. A broken anesthetic carpule is only considered a sharps item if it is broken, otherwise it can be discarded in the regular trash.

28. Which of the following is not true regarding hand washing?

    c. Hands do not have to be dried completely before donning gloves – Hands should be dried as completely as possible before donning gloves. Moisture retained on your hands and the warmth generated by wearing the gloves can lead to bacteria developing under nails and in between fingers.

29. Nitrile utility gloves are used for

    d. all of the above – Nitrile utility gloves are worn for all of the above. They are never worn to treat patients.

30. How often should the suction lines be flushed with an EPA-approved solution?

    a. daily – Suction lines should be flushed daily and sometimes more than once a day depending, on how much treatment you perform that results in patient bleeding and fluid generation.

31. All of the following are disposed of in the sharps container except

    b. intact anesthetic carpules – Contrary to popular practice, these do not need to be disposed of in the sharps container unless they are broken, shattered, or have blood in them. Otherwise, they can go into the regular lab trash.

32. Using an EPA-approved solution, cold sterilization can be achieved by

    b. 6 hours of exposure to instruments.

33. All of the following reasons are true for using a dental dam except

    c. to maintain patient airway – This is not a reason for using a dental dam.

34. When using the chemclave, all except the following must be achieved for sterilization to be successful:

    d. recommended cassettes are used – The type of cassette has no bearing on achieving sterilization.

35. High-level chemical germicides are registered

    a. as sterilants/disinfectants – The EPA considers high-level germicides sterilants/disinfectants.

36. Single-use instruments

    d. are designed to be used only one time and then discarded – Items such as saliva ejectors and prophy angles are examples of single-use items. They are NOT to be cleaned and reused due to their design and durability and difficulty with thoroughly cleaning and sterilizing.

37. Lab cases such as dentures or partials should be

    d. all of the above – Lab cases should be handled like any other item and safely disinfected prior to placing in the patient's mouth or sending out of the office for processing. They have the same infectious potential as any other item that the dental health care worker may come into contact with.

38. When recapping an anesthetic needle, OSHA protocol recommends

    a. using a recapping device – Using a recapping device is designed to protect the dental health care worker from needlestick and should be used with every patient. The other methods listed are done but are not the safest methods.

39. Droplet infection can be best described as

    a. occurring with inhalation of aerosol generated during dental procedures.

40. The most common mode of disease transmission that occurs in the dental office is

    c. direct or indirect.

41. Instruments considered "critical" should always

    c. be sterilized.

42. Sepsis can be best defined as

    c. the presence of disease-producing microorganisms.

43. Steam sterilization under pressure can be achieved using a/an

    b. autoclave.

44. Semicritical instruments

    d. all of the above – Semicritical items do not penetrate soft tissue, contact soft oral tissue, and require sterilization.

45. Bloody gauze or tissue must be disposed by

    b. placing in the biohazard waste.

46. The best way to manage a mercury spill is to

    d. use a mercury spill kit.

47. Discarded scrap amalgam is best stored by

    d. storing it under water or fixer in a sealed container.

48. Ultrasonic cleaners are available as

    d. all of the above – Liquids, enzymatic and nonenzymatic formulations, and nonenzymatic effervescing soluble tablets are all types of ultrasonic cleaning solutions.

49. The preferred method for cleaning hard surfaces would be

    c. disposable toweling and an EPA-registered disinfectant for hard surfaces.

50. Mask selection should be based on

    d. all of the above – Level of protection, fit, and breathability should all be factors to consider when choosing a facemask.

51. Prior to surgical procedures, hand hygiene must be performed with

    a. antimicrobial soap and water with aggressive rubbing.

52. In the dental office, the best way to reduce the risk of contracting a communicable disease is to

    d. all of the above – Taking a thorough health history, using disposable items, and wearing personal protective equipment are all steps to take to reduce the risk of contracting a communicable disease.

53. The ultrasonic cleaner contains a liquid medium to aid in the removal of debris from instruments. The solution should be changed

    a. at the end of the day.

54. Which chemical agent is acceptable for clinical contact surface disinfection?

    a. EPA-registered

55. Critical instruments are considered

    a. to contact and penetrate tissues.

56. A curing light emits a visible light, so it is imperative that you wear

    c. protective tinted eyewear.

57. Dental handpieces (both high and slow speed) should be sterilized

    b. after each patient.

58. Why is it important to dry instrument packages inside the sterilizer after the end of the sterilization cycle?

    a. It prevents microbes from penetrating the moist package. – Moist packages can introduce microbes into the pouches and cause contamination.

59. When is the most appropriate time to use an alcohol-based hand rub?

    d. only when there is no visible soil on the hands

60. Some patient-care instruments and armamentarium such as blood pressure cuffs, stethoscope, and pulse oximeter are categorized as

    c. noncritical – These items do not touch soft tissue or mucous membranes and are not exposed to saliva or blood.

61. Instruments are sterilized by chemical sterilization for how many minutes at what temperature?

    a. 10 to 20/250 – 10 to 20 minutes at 250 degrees F.

62. Plastic disposable items are designed to be

    c. discarded even if placed on instrument tray and not used.

63. When using the dry-heat sterilization method, instruments must be dried completely to avoid

    c. rusting.

64. A steam sterilizer requires which kind of solution?

    d. distilled water – Using distilled water prevents mineral buildup within the sterilizer.

65. To "flash autoclave" an instrument, the following must be done:

    a. 8 minutes for a wrapped load at 250 degrees F at 30 psi

66. Dry-heat sterilization requires how many hours for sterilization?

    c. 8 to10

67. Biological indicators used to test steam sterilizers contain

    a. *bacillus stearothermophilus*.

68. Ethylene oxide is a form of gas sterilization that requires approximately how many hours of exposure to be effective?

    c. 10–16

69. To avoid cross-contamination from patient to patient, it is recommended that you do the following:

    b. Clean the dental chair and bracket table between patients – This is the only scenario out of the four that could potentially create a patient-to-patient contamination scenario.

70. The fiber-optic light surface on the high-speed handpiece should be cleaned with isopropyl alcohol and a cotton tip applicator

    c. after it is sterilized – Oftentimes, after sterilization the fiber-optic light cover will have a haze and is best cleaned with isopropyl alcohol.

71. This method of sterilization requires that items must be completely submerged and undisturbed for at least 6 hours for cold sterilization.

    d. glutaraldehyde

72. When using a chemclave, which liquid product is used during the sterilization process?

    a. deodorized alcohol formaldehyde

73. A negative sporicidal test you run on the autoclave comes back as negative. What does this mean?

    a. Sterilization did occur.

74. Adequate ventilation is required for which sterilizer?

    b. chemclave – The gas vapors that are given off are considered cancer causing, and ventilation is key when using this type of sterilizer.

75. The type of gloves used during disinfection and clean up procedures are called

    d. utility gloves.

Section III: Occupational Safety

This topic of the Infection Control portion of the Certified Dental Assisting Examination consists of 30% or 30 of the 100 multiple-choice items. The questions related to this section of the Infection Control Examination are based upon your knowledge of the following:

- Follow the standards and guidelines of occupational safety for dental office personnel.
- Incorporate all safety measures when using chemical and physical hazards.
- Maintain and document a quality-assurance (quality-improvement) program for infection control and safety throughout the dental office.

Key Terms

blood-borne pathogens – disease-spreading organisms found in the blood that can be passed on by contact with the blood of an infected individual

contaminated laundry – any item of clothing that has been splattered with biological waste materials or hazardous chemicals

contaminated sharps – any piece of equipment that is capable of causing a break in the skin that has been exposed to biohazard materials such as needles

engineering controls – regulations intended to reduce the risk of infection due to sharp materials contaminated with biohazard waste

exposure incident – any workplace event in which an employee has been exposed to a hazardous material and is at increased risk of infection as a result

occupational exposure – any reasonably anticipated exposure to secretions of the eye, mucosa, skin, parenteral, or any contact with blood or saliva that may be a result of employment tasks

parenteral – access directly to the bloodstream; a cut, puncture, needlestick

regulated waste – liquid or semiliquid blood or other potentially infectious materials or items contaminated with blood that would release these substances in a liquid or semiliquid state if compressed and sharp

sharps – objects that can penetrate a worker's skin, such as needles, scalpels, broken glass, capillary tubes and ends of dental wires

Universal Precautions – guidelines established by the CDC to help protect health care workers and patients from the transmission of infectious diseases

Work Practice Control – regulations and standards that are employed to help reduce employee health risks while on the job

Quick Review Outline

A. The dental assistant should be familiar with the Standards and Guidelines of Occupational Safety for dental office personnel.

1. The OSHA Bloodborne Pathogens Standard, which became effective March 1992, requires that every employer perform a workplace exposure determination in order to identify hazards such as exposure to blood and other potentially infectious materials and implement appropriate controls to minimize patient exposure.

2. In 2001, "engineering controls" became part of the standard and add language to the definition section of the original 1991 standard that reflects the development over the last decade in the use of safer medical devices such as scalpel blades, anesthetic needles, and other sharp items in an effort to reduce or eliminate employee exposure.

3. Occupational Safety and Health Administration (OSHA) Hazard Communication Standard is set up so that the employee has the proper information and training on handling hazardous materials in the office. Employees should be trained in the proper handling of hazardous chemicals and other materials used in the

dental office. Employees must be trained in the first 30 days of employment on the proper handling of hazardous materials and the correct attire or personal protective equipment that must be worn when handling these materials and then annually thereafter.

   a. The key items that should be covered in the Hazard Communication Standard orientation should include the following:

      i. an overall explanation of OSHA laws and how they apply to employees

      ii. explanation of the epidemiology and symptoms of HBV and HIV/AIDS

      iii. discussion about who is at risk in the dental office

      iv. transmission modes of different microorganisms

      v. methods of infection control in the workplace

      vi. review of Universal/Standard Precautions

      vii. personal protective equipment and its use

      viii. review of proper hand washing techniques for various situations

      ix. how hazardous materials spills are to be cleaned

      x. postexposure incident procedure

      xi. coverage of the Hazardous Communication Standard

      xii. chemical labels and how to read them

      xiii. how to read and interpret an SDS sheet

      xiv. proper storage of chemicals and how they are inventoried

      xv. hazardous waste laws and how to comply with those laws

      xvi. how to use sharps containers

      xvii. who in the office is responsible for maintaining records and how those records are to be maintained

      xviii. review of medical consent forms

      xix. familiarization with HBV forms

      xx. what engineering control records are and how they are kept

      xxi. Safety training certifications and when training is to take place

4. Understanding the proper first aid procedures when there is an exposure as described in the OSHA Bloodborne Pathogens and Hazard Communication Standards

   a. Every employee should have a valid, up-to-date CPR certification.

   b. The office must possess a fully functioning oxygen tank with a positive-pressure mask (sterile), and the equipment should be charged and checked on a regular basis.

   c. A listing of the nearest fire department, ambulance, emergency room, and police department should be posted in plain view for all employees to refer to.

   d. Charged fire extinguishers must be placed throughout the office and in plain view for employees to use. Training on how to use these extinguishers must be provided on a yearly basis.

   e. A stocked first aid kit must be placed in plain view for all employees to have access to it. Replenish kits as needed.

   f. Ideally, an automated external defibrillator should be available, and personnel should be trained on how to use it.

   g. Employee training on responding to puncture wounds, burns, eye injury, chemical burns, and other non–life-threatening emergencies should be provided on an annual basis.

   h. A fully functioning eye-wash station must be available in the event there is an exposure.

   i. Sharps containers, syringe/needle recapping devices, and scalpel blade removal systems should be in place to prevent puncture wounds.

   j. Chemicals should be clearly labeled, and first aid instruction on what to do in case of exposure should be covered.

   k. Signage indicating radiation, hot objects such as sterilizers, and other areas considered dangerous must be clearly labeled.

   l. A posted evacuation plan must be in plain view for all employees to use in the event there is an emergency that requires evacuation of employees from the workplace.

B. The dental assistant should be able to demonstrate safety measures when using chemical and physical hazards.

   1. Listed below are some of the chemicals and/or hazards the dental assistant may encounter in the workplace.

      a. mercury – As mentioned previously, this metal is liquid at room temperature and should never be touched with bare hands. It is toxic, and if there is a spill, proper cleanup using a mercury spill kit should be used. Long-term exposure to mercury can cause a host of health problems. Fortunately, most offices do not use mercury in its raw form but instead use premeasured capsules. Alloy contains mercury, and scrap alloy should be stored in a jar with a screw-top lid under fixer or mineral oil and then picked up or disposed of in conjunction with the EPA laws of your state. If an employee demonstrates mercury poisoning, a urine test can be done to confirm any suspicion.

      b. nitrous oxide (N_2O_2) – A mixture of nitrogen and oxygen renders a gas called nitrous oxide. Nitrous oxide provides an analgesic and light sedation effect for most patients. NEVER leave a patient unattended while he/she is under the influence of nitrous oxide, and always watch for signs of responsiveness such as ongoing dialogue and the movement of the reservoir bag. A patient should never become unconscious or fall asleep while exposed to nitrous oxide. The patient should always be able to take commands and respond to questions when asked. If a patient becomes unresponsive, let the operator know so the mixture can be adjusted. If a patient becomes agitated or unconscious and you are unable to rouse the patient, shut the nitrous off and give them 100% oxygen immediately. Leave the patient in the supine position until he or she becomes conscious and responsive. If the patient does not become conscious, maintain an airway, administer oxygen, call 911, and monitor for possible CPR administration. Proper titration of N_2O_2 gases must be performed to ensure the safety of your patient. Regardless of which delivery unit your office uses (portable or wall mounted), there should be a proper scavenger system, and the equipment should be checked and tested on a regular basis to ensure that it is working properly.

> **NOTE** If you are pregnant or trying to become pregnant, do not assist with procedures that involve the use of nitrous oxide. Patients who are pregnant or trying to become pregnant should not elect the use of nitrous oxide. Nitrous oxide has been proven to cause spontaneous miscarriages and damage to the unborn fetus and can impede fertility for those trying to conceive.

      c. caustic agents – Some chemicals used in the dental field can be considered caustic. Proper protective equipment should be used when handling these materials, and the employee should have the proper training if an exposure occurs. All chemicals should be labeled, and a binder containing SDS sheets should be available to all employees in the event there is an exposure.

      d. airborne particles and contaminants – Airborne particles and contaminants are always present in the dental field. Proper protective equipment such as goggles, masks, and face shields should be available to the employee and worn when there is a potential for exposure to these contaminants. Contaminants such as blood, saliva, and microorganisms can become aerosolized and can be inhaled by the dental assistant. Also, flying debris while delivering dental treatment can pose a risk for eye injury to the patient and the dental assistant.

      e. bonding materials – Bonding materials can contain chemicals that can chemically burn the skin upon contact. Etchant, which is usually blue or clear and is used to remove the smear layer from the enamel of the tooth, can cause minor surface burns when coming into contact with oral tissues and skin. Immediately rinse with water until all traces of the chemical are removed.

      f. curing light – When using the curing light, protective glasses must be worn by both the operator and the assistant. Glasses must also be provided to the patient. These glasses must meet safety standards to shield against the exposure of visible light. Long-term exposure to visible light from the curing light can cause permanent vision damage.

      g. lasers – Protective eyewear is mandatory for both the operator and patient.

      h. latex – A small portion of the population is allergic to latex. Allergic reactions can range from an itchy rash to full-blown anaphylactic shock, which, if not treated immediately, can lead to death. If your patient expresses any type of allergic reaction to latex, DO NOT take a chance! Use vinyl or other non-latex gloves during any contact with the patient (also make sure that other rubber items are latex free, such as prophy angles and saliva ejectors). If you use latex gloves on your patient and the patient begins to exhibit an allergic reaction, proper first aid and follow-up medical care should be delivered. Your doctor should administer the proper medications, and you should call 911 and retrieve and set up the oxygen tank and mask and assist with maintaining the patient's airway until medical help arrives. As an operator, if you are allergic to latex, make sure your doctor provides appropriate gloves for you to wear when assisting and carrying out your daily routine duties.

C. Maintaining and documenting a quality-assurance program for infection control and safety

1. Bloodborne Pathogens Standard. This standard was initiated as a quality-assurance measure to provide protection to all health care workers who come in contact with blood, saliva, or other body fluids in the course of providing dental treatment. The standard includes:
   a. personal protective equipment or universal precautions
   b. establishment of engineering/work practice controls
   c. housekeeping
   d. proper handling of infectious waste
   e. maintaining employee work records
   f. written exposure control plan that is in place
   g. providing the hepatitis B vaccine series to all employees with occupational exposure
   h. providing information and training to workers
   i. maintaining worker medical training records
   j. using labels and signage to communicate hazards at work

2. Engineering and Work Practice Controls – These **engineering controls** help eliminate the possibility of the employee being injured. Special containers for disposing of contaminated needles, blades, broken glass, instruments, or other "sharp" items are **work practice controls**.
   A. dental dams
   B. high-speed evacuators
   C. Sharps containers
   D. needle-recapping devices
   E. biohazard bags or containers for potentially infectious materials

3. Waste Handling
   a. Handling waste is a daily activity in the dental office. **Regulated waste** is defined as liquid or semiliquid blood or other potentially infectious materials or items contaminated with blood that would release these substances in a liquid or semiliquid state if compressed and sharp, which are objects that can penetrate a worker's skin, such as needles, scalpels, broken glass, capillary tubes and ends of dental wires. Other items that may be caked with dried blood and are capable of releasing infectious waste during handling are also considered biohazard waste.
   b. Prompt disposal of sharps in a container that is readily accessible to the location where the sharps was used. They must be puncture resistant and leakproof and sealed before being picked up or shipped for disposal.
   c. Bloody gauze or other items contaminated with blood must be disposed of in a red bag labeled with the biohazard emblem. These bags are picked up by a licensed hauler.

4. Housekeeping and Laundry
   a. There should be a written plan and schedule for cleaning up each area where exposures occur. The different methods of decontaminating different surfaces must be specified, determined by the type of surface to be cleaned. For example, you would clean up a blood spill differently on carpet than on tile flooring. Employees should clean:
      i. when surfaces are obviously contaminated;
      ii. after any spill;
      iii. at the end of the work shift.

When there is no exposure of blood or saliva, decontamination is not required, but sanitizing the room is recommended. For example, after taking radiographs, sanitizing the equipment is necessary, but decontaminating the floors and walls is not required. However, an extraction that generated the aerosolization of blood and saliva with a high-speed handpiece would require complete decontamination of the entire room. If surfaces draped with protective coverings come into contact with blood or saliva, the coverings must be changed as soon as the procedure is completed and during the decontamination process.

5. Record keeping is mandatory, and medical and training records are essential to maintain when running a dental office.
   a. Medical records must be established for all employees who might be exposed to an occupational hazard. Records are always kept confidential.
   b. Records contain such items as hepatitis B vaccination status, occupational exposure incidents, and refusal of any recommended vaccinations.
   c. These medical records must be kept 30 years past the last date of employment of the employee.
   d. Training records are documented records that indicate dates of training, the trainer's name, and their qualifications. They are to be kept for at least 3 years and must be transferred to the new owner should the dentist sell his/her practice.

6. Exposure Control Plan
   a. A written exposure plan must include identification of job classifications and tasks.
   b. It must be accessible to all employees and updated at least every year.
   c. It provides a schedule of how and when the standard will be implemented and includes schedules and methods for communication of hazards to employees.
   d. It provides procedures for evaluating the circumstances of an exposure incident and should include provisions that are designed to maintain the privacy of those employees who have had an exposure.

7. When an Exposure Incident Occurs
   a. Employees should report an exposure incident to their employer as soon as possible.
   b. Follow-up must be made with the employee who was exposed.
   c. The employer must provide the attending health care professional with all pertinent information such as the route of exposure, what type of exposure, employee medical records, and any other information that may be needed in treating the employee.
   d. The health care provider must provide the employer with a written opinion that the employee has been counseled on the results. All other information is strictly confidential.

8. The employer is responsible for the development, implementation, and maintenance of the written hazard communication program. Some of those components of the hazard communication program are:
   a. inventory of chemicals
   b. ensure containers are labeled
   c. obtain SDS available to workers
   d. conduct training of workers on how to read MSDS sheets
   e. identify a coordinator of the office program
   f. keep records of all training and information provided to employees

9. Hazard Communication Standard. This standard was constructed to protect all workers who may come in contact with potential injuries and illnesses from an exposure to any hazardous chemicals in the work-place. This would include chemicals that can cause skin burns, lung damage, and flammability. Some of the requirements include:
   a. Safety Data Sheets (SDS)
   b. labeling
   c. record keeping
   d. Written Hazard Communication Program
   e. Employees who may be exposed to hazardous chemicals must have a written hazard communication program.

10. OSHA Task Organization
   a. OSHA categorizes tasks in order of potential exposure to contaminated blood, body fluids, or tissues.
      i. Category 1 – Employees in this category are classified as dentists, hygienists, assistants, and laboratory technicians.
      ii. Category 2 – Tasks that have no exposure to blood, body fluids, or tissues but may have an unplanned exposure to Category 1 tasks. Employees classified in this category may include clerical or nonprofessional workers.
      iii. Category 3 – Tasks that have no exposure to blood, body fluids, or tissues. Employees classified in this category may include receptionists, bookkeepers, and insurance clerks.

Scope and Application
• The Standard applies to all occupational exposure to blood and other potentially infectious materials (OPIMs) and includes part-time employees, designated first aiders, and mental health workers, as well as exposed medical personnel. • OPIMs include saliva in dental procedures, cerebrospinal fluid, unfixed tissue, semen, vaginal secretions, and body fluids visibly contaminated with blood.

Methods of Compliance
• General—Standard precautions. • Engineering and work practice controls. • Personal protective equipment. • Housekeeping.

Standard Precautions
• *All* human blood and OPIMs are considered infectious. • The *same* precautions must be taken with all blood and OPIMs.

Engineering Controls
• Whenever feasible, engineering controls must be the primary method for controlling exposure. • Examples include needleless IVs, self-sheathing needles, sharps disposal containers, covered centrifuge buckets, aerosol-free tubes, and leak-proof containers. • Engineering controls must be evaluated and documented regularly.

Sharps Containers
• Readily accessible and as close as practical to work area. • Puncture resistant. • Labeled or color coded. • Leak proof. • Closeable. • *Routinely replaced* so there is no overflow.

Work Practice Controls
• Handwashing following glove removal. • No recapping, breaking, or bending of needles. • No eating, drinking, smoking, and so on in work area. • No storage of food or drink where blood or OPIMs are stored. • Minimize splashing, splattering of blood, and splashing of OPIMs. • No mouth pipetting. • Specimens must be transported in leak-proof, labeled containers. They must be placed in a secondary container if outside contamination of primary container occurs. • Equipment must be decontaminated before servicing or shipping. Areas that cannot be decontaminated must be labeled.

Figure 3-6 (Continues)

(Continued)

Personal Protective Equipment

- Includes eye protection, gloves, protective clothing, and resuscitation equipment.
- Must be readily accessible and employers must require their use.
- Must be stored at work site.

Eye Protection

- Is required whenever there is potential for splashing, spraying, or splattering to the eyes or mucous membranes.
- If necessary, use eye protection with a mask, or use a chin-length face shield.
- Prescription glasses may be fitted with solid side shields.
- Decontamination procedures must be developed.

Gloves

- Must be worn whenever hand contact with blood, OPIMs, mucous membranes, non-intact skin, or contaminated surfaces/items or when performing vascular access procedures (phlebotomy).
- Type required:
    —Vinyl or latex for general use.
    —Alternatives must be available if employee has allergic reactions (e.g., powderless).
    —Utility gloves for surface disinfection.
    —Puncture resistant when handling sharps (e.g., Central Supply).

Protective Clothing

- Must be worn whenever splashing or splattering to skin or clothing may occur.
- Type required depends on exposure. Prevention of skin and clothes contamination is the key.
- Examples:
    —Low-level-exposure lab coats.
    —Moderate-level-exposure, fluid-resistant gown.
    —High-level-exposure, fluid-proof apron, head and foot covering.
- *Note:* If personal protective equipment (PPE) is considered protective clothing, then the *employer must launder it*.

Housekeeping

- There must be a written schedule for cleaning and disinfection.
- Contaminated equipment and surfaces must be cleaned as soon as feasible for obvious contamination or at end of work shift if no contamination has occurred.
- Protective coverings may be used over equipment.

Regulated Waste Containers (Non-Sharp)

- Closeable.
- Leak proof.
- Labeled or color coded.
- Placed in secondary container if outside of container is contaminated.

Laundry

- Handled as little as possible.
- Bagged at location of use.
- Labeled or color coded.
- Transported in bags that prevent soak-through or leakage.

Figure 3-6 (Continues)

Laundry Facility

- Two options:
  1. Standard precautions for all laundry (alternative color coding allowed if recognized).
  2. Precautions only for contaminated laundry (must be red bagged or biohazard labeled).
- Laundry personnel must use PPE and have a sharps container accessible.

Hepatitis B Vaccination

- Made available within 10 days to all employees with occupational exposure.
- Free to employees.
- May be required for student to be admitted to a college health program, as well as to an externship.
- Given according to U.S. Public Health Service guidelines.
- Employee must first be evaluated by a health care professional.
- Health care professional gives a written opinion.
- If the vaccine is refused, the employee signs a declination form.
- Vaccine must be available later if initially refused.

Postexposure Follow-up

- Wash thoroughly with antimicrobial soap.
- Have a blood draw as soon as possible or within 2 hours.
- Document exposure incident.
- Identify source individual (if possible).
- Attempt to test source if consent is obtained.
- Provide results to the exposed employee.

Labels

- Biohazard symbol and word *Biohazard* must be visible.
- Fluorescent orange/orange-red with contrasting letters may also be used.
- Red bags/containers may be substituted for labels.
- Labels are required on:
  —Regulated waste.
  —Refrigerators/freezers with blood of OPIMs.
  —Transport/storage containers.
  —Contaminated equipment.

Information and Training

- Required for all employees with occupational exposure.
- Training required initially, annually, and if there are new procedures.
- Training material must be appropriate for the employees' literacy and education levels.
- Training must be interactive and allow for questions and answers.

Training Components

- Modes of HIV/HBV transmission.
- Explanation of exposure control plan.
- Explanation of engineering, work practice controls.
- Explanation of blood-borne standard.
- Epidemiology and symptoms of blood-borne disease.
- How to select the proper PPE.
- How to decontaminate equipment, surfaces, and so on.
- Information about hepatitis B vaccine.
- Postexposure follow-up procedures.
- Label/color code system.

Figure 3-6 (Continues)

(Continued)

Medical Records
Records must be kept for each employee with occupational exposure and include: • A copy of employee's vaccination status and date. • A copy of postexposure follow-up evaluation procedures. • Health care professional's written opinions. • Confidentiality must be maintained. • Records must be maintained for 30 years, plus the duration of employment.

Training Records
Records are kept for 3 years from date of training and include: • Date of training. • Summary of contents of training program. • Name and qualifications of trainer. • Names and job titles of all persons attending.

Exposure Control Plan Components
• A written plan for each workplace with occupational exposure. • Written policies/procedures for complying with the standard. • A cohesive document or a guiding document referencing existing policies/procedures.

Exposure Control Plan
• A list of job classifications where occupational exposure control occurs (e.g., medical assistant, clinical laboratory scientist, dental hygienist). • A list of tasks where exposure occurs (e.g., medical assistant who performs venipuncture). • Methods/policies/procedures for compliance. • Procedures for sharps disposal. • Disinfection policies/procedures. • Procedures for selection of PPE. • Regulated waste disposal procedures. • Laundry procedures. • Hepatitis B vaccination procedures. • Postexposure follow-up procedures. • Training procedures. • Plan must be accessible to employees and be updated annually.

Employee Responsibilities
• Go through training and cooperate. • Obey policies. • Use universal precaution techniques. • Use PPE. • Use safe work practices. • Use engineering controls.

Employee Responsibilities

• Report unsafe work conditions to employer.
• Maintain clean work areas.
   Cooperation between employer and employees regarding the Standard will facilitate understanding of the law, thereby benefiting all persons who are exposed to HIV, HBV, and OPIMs by minimizing the risk of exposure to pathogens.
   Meeting the OSHA standard is not optional, and failure to comply can result in a fine that may total $10,000 for each employee.

Figure 3-6 Understanding OSHA's blood-borne/hazardous materials standard.

Important Information You Should Know

1. Understand the OSHA Bloodborne Pathogens Standard.
2. Understand the OSHA Hazard Communication Standard.
3. Know how to perform appropriate first aid procedures.
4. Understand the importance of documenting and reporting all exposures such as puncture wounds, needle-sticks, or chemical exposures.
5. Understand how to incorporate all safety measures when using chemical and physical hazards in the dental field.
6. Understand the importance of maintaining and documenting a quality-assurance program for infection control and safety.

Study Checklist

1. Review text on infection control.
2. Understand the government agencies such as OSHA and the CDC and their role in infection control in the dental field.
3. Review OSHA Hazard Communication and Blood Borne Pathogens Standard for the dental field.
4. Review terminology as it relates to infection control.

Section III: Occupational Safety – Review Questions

Use the Answer Sheet found in Appendix A.

1. The OSHA standard states that employee exposure incident records are to be
   a. entered into the computer employee database.
   b. faxed to the employee's physician.
   c. kept on file for 30 days.
   d. kept confidential and filed in the employee's medical record.

2. When working with a visible light-cure unit,
   a. the dental unit light must be turned to the off position.
   b. a face shield must be worn.
   c. protective visible-light eyewear is required.
   d. protective eyewear is not necessary.

3. The written Hazard Communication program contains all the following except
   a. SDS information.
   b. laundry schedule.
   c. hazardous chemicals log.
   d. employee training records.

4. Employees should have training on using a fire extinguisher
   a. only after there has been a fire.
   b. once a year.
   c. twice a year.
   d. only the DDS needs to be trained.

5. The first aid kit should be
   a. out in plain sight in the event you may need it.
   b. updated and accessible to all employees.
   c. only accessible to the DDS because it contains medications.
   d. stored in a cool, dark place so the contents will be preserved.

6. A fully charged oxygen tank with _____ should be accessible.
   a. a clean and disinfected mask
   b. a positive-pressure mask
   c. an ambu bag
   d. an expiration tag

7. Which documentation should be included with all hazardous and nonhazardous chemicals found in the dental office?
   a. SDS sheet
   b. sharps log
   c. sterilization log
   d. employee training records

8. An exposure-control plan is
   a. a written plan to eliminate or minimize occupational exposures.
   b. a written plan that directs you in what to do if there is a medical emergency.
   c. a set of directives for disposing of hazardous chemicals.
   d. a log that is kept when there is a workplace injury.

9. The employer must provide the hepatitis B series to an employee
   a. the day of employment.
   b. within 10 days of employment.
   c. within 1 year of employment.
   d. only if there has been an exposure to the virus.

10. An **exposure incident** is considered
    a. when eye, mouth, or other mucous membrane or nonintact skin comes into contact with blood or saliva.
    b. when there is a procedure that presents a potential for exposure.
    c. when the patient comes into contact with a contaminant at the office.
    d. something that usually does not happen with proper training.

11. Worker medical and training records can be shared with
    a. the employee's family.
    b. the office manager.
    c. only the employee.
    d. nobody; they are confidential.

12. During the administration of nitrous oxide, the assistant should
    a. monitor the patient for breathing and response.
    b. never leave the patient unattended.
    c. do a complete review of the patient's medical history prior to the procedure.
    d. all of the above.

13. If the operatory was used only for an exam, it would be necessary to
    a. decontaminate the entire room; the patient may have HIV.
    b. change only the barriers that were touched by the operator and patient.
    c. wipe down all surfaces of the room with an EPA-approved disinfectant.
    d. do nothing; it did not generate blood or saliva droplets.

14. OSHA standards regarding contaminated laundry include all of the following EXCEPT:
    a. A washer and dryer may be used on site.
    b. Employee training is not required to do a load of lab jackets.
    c. It must be handled as little as possible.
    d. Laundry transport bags must be identified with a biohazard symbol.

15. Regulated waste is identified as
    a. flammable materials.
    b. soiled laundry.
    c. disposables.
    d. blood-soaked gauze, uncapped needles, and infectious materials.

16. Methods of reducing hazards in the dental office include all of the following EXCEPT
    a. washing hands before and after donning gloves.
    b. making available a functional fire extinguisher.
    c. maintaining adequate ventilation in the office.
    d. helping the patient remain calm during the dental procedure.

17. The best way to recap a needle is to
    a. let the DDS do it.
    b. bend it in half and then put in the sharps container.
    c. use a needle-recapping device.
    d. leave the needle on the tray and dispose of it after the procedure.

18. You are treating a patient with a history of latex allergy. The alternative to using latex gloves would be which type of glove?
    a. nitrile
    b. vinyl
    c. plastic
    d. rubber

19. During an amalgam procedure, the amalgam does not mix with the mercury, and you have a mercury exposure. To clean up the mercury exposure, you would do which of the following?
    a. Vacuum it up with the HVE.
    b. Pick it up with gloved hands and dispose it into the commode.
    c. Use a mercury spill kit.
    d. Call a biohazard specialist to come in and clean up the spill.

20. According to the Occupational Safety and Health Administration (OSHA), an **occupational exposure** is defined as a(an)
    a. latent radiographic exposure.
    b. occupational emergency.
    c. needlestick or puncture from an instrument.
    d. use of the eyewash station after a chemical substance enters the eyes.

21. How is the Bloodborne Pathogens Standard best described?
    a. Follow the same infection-control procedure for all types of health care facilities
    b. Blood is always considered infectious.
    c. Only use infection-control procedures approved by OSHA.
    d. All patient blood and body fluids are potentially infectious.

22. OSHA is an acronym for the following:
    a. Occupational Safety and Health Agency
    b. Occupational Safety and Health Administration
    c. Occupational Sterilization and Hazard Administration
    d. Organization of the Safety and Health Agency

23. exposure-control plan should be
    a. accessible to each employee.
    b. reviewed and updated on an annual basis.
    c. a written protocol for the office.
    d. all of the above.

24. When an employee has a needlestick injury, the employee should
    a. accept blood testing for HIV and Hat recommended intervals.
    b. have the HBV gamma globulin administered as soon as possible.
    c. document the incident with the office manager.
    d. all of the above.

25. Part of the hazard communication protocol includes
    a. designating a safety coordinator for the office.
    b. keeping an MSDS book available for all employees to reference.
    c. keeping a list of hazardous chemicals and their quantity with their locations disclosed.
    d. all of the above.

26. According to the American Heart Association, cardiopulmonary resuscitation certification should be updated
    a. every year.
    b. every 2 years.
    c. every 18 weeks.
    d. only when the guidelines change.

27. OSHA considers Category 1 workers as those who
    a. handle laboratory items.
    b. handle charts and paperwork.
    c. perform general housekeeping duties.
    d. come into contact with blood and body fluids or tissues.

28. OSHA states that Category 3 workers
    a. are not exposed to blood or bodily fluids.
    b. are exposed to blood only.
    c. are exposed to hazardous chemicals.
    d. none of the above.

29. After an exposure incident, according to the blood-borne pathogens standard, an employer must keep a log that includes
    a. location of the incident (where in the office it happened).
    b. description of how the incident occurred.
    c. what type of follow-up care was taken after the incident.
    d. all of the above.

30. According to OSHA, employee training records relating to the Bloodborne and Hazard Communication Standard must be maintained for a minimum of
    a. 6 months.
    b. 1 year.
    c. 3 years.
    d. 30 years.

31. Who provides the SDS sheets that are required to be kept in the dental office?
    a. employer
    b. office manager
    c. chemical manufacturer
    d. OSHA

32. The letters CDC stand for
    a. Centers for Disease Criteria.
    b. Center for Dental Cleanliness.
    c. Center for Dental Chemicals.
    d. Centers for Disease Control.

33. The standard that is created to protect employees against occupational exposure to blood-borne, disease-causing organisms is referred to as which standard?
    a. OSHA Bloodborne Pathogens Standard
    b. Environmental Protection Standard
    c. Centers for Disease Control Standard
    d. Food and Drug Administration Standard

34. Which of the following is a work practice control?
    a. hand washing following glove removal
    b. sharps disposal containers
    c. ventilation hoods
    d. eye-wash stations

35. Which of the following is an engineering control?
    a. hand washing after glove removal
    b. self-sheathing needles
    c. no storage of food or drink in the work area
    d. no mouth pipetting

Section III:
Occupational Safety –
Answers and Rationales

1. The OSHA standard states that employee exposure incident records are to be

    d. kept confidential and filed in the employee's medical record – These results are confidential, and it is up to the employee to decide whether they want to share this information with their employer. They are not required to do so.

2. When working with a visible light-cure unit,

    c. protective visible light eyewear is required.

3. The written hazard communication program contains all the following except

    b. laundry schedule.

4. Employees should have training on using a fire extinguisher

    b. once a year.

5. The first aid kit should be

    b. updated and accessible to all employees.

6. A fully charged oxygen tank with _____ should be accessible.

    b. a positive-pressure mask

7. Which documentation should be included with all hazardous and nonhazardous chemicals found in the dental office?

    a. SDS sheet – This is intended to provide workers and emergency personnel with procedures for handling or working with that substance in a safe manner. It includes information such as physical data on melting point, boiling point, flash point, toxicity, health effects, first aid, reactivity, storage, disposal, protective equipment, and spill-handling procedures.

8. An exposure-control plan is

    a. written plan to eliminate or minimize occupational exposures – This plan is a compilation of standard operating procedures that define infection-control practices, reducing exposure, and methods of implementation.

9. The employer must provide the hepatitis B series to an employee

    b. within days of employment.

10. An exposure incident is considered

    a. when eye, mouth, or other mucous membrane or nonintact skin comes into contact with blood or saliva.

11. Worker medical and training records can be shared with

    b. the office manager – These records are not necessarily confidential, and the office manager usually has access to them.

12. During the administration of nitrous oxide, the assistant should

    d. all of the above.

13. If the operatory was used only for an exam, it would be necessary to

    c. wipe down all surfaces of the room with an EPA-approved disinfectant – Since the generation of blood, saliva, or other fluids did not occur, simply disinfecting the room is adequate.

14. OSHA standards regarding contaminated laundry include all of the following EXCEPT:

    b. Employee training is not required to do a load of lab jackets. – Special training is not required to wash a load of lab jackets, although protocol should be established such as the use of hot water, soap, and bleach.

15. Regulated waste is identified as

    d. blood-soaked gauze, uncapped needles, and infectious materials.

16. Methods of reducing hazards in the dental office include all of the following EXCEPT

    d. helping the patient remain calm during the dental procedure – This is not part of reducing hazards in the office but instead is part of helping your patients be comfortable during their visit.

17. The best way to recap a needle is to

    c. use a needle-recapping device.

18. You are treating a patient with a history of latex allergy. The alternative to using latex gloves would be which type of glove?

    b. Vinyl – Vinyl gloves are the best and most often used alternative to latex gloves. Nitrile gloves are too thick, plastic is too thin, and rubber is not advised.

19. During an amalgam procedure, the amalgam does not mix with the mercury and you have a mercury exposure. To clean up the mercury exposure, you would do which of the following?

    c. Use a mercury spill kit.

20. According to the Occupational Safety and Health Administration (OSHA), an occupational exposure is defined as a(an)

   c. **needlestick or puncture from an instrument.**

21. How is the Bloodborne Pathogens Standard best described?

   d. **All patient blood and body fluids are potentially infectious.**

22. OSHA is an acronym for the following:

   b. **Occupational Safety and Health Administration – This is a federally controlled entity that is concerned with worker safety, not patient safety.**

23. An exposure-control plan should be

   d. **all of the above – An exposure plan should be accessible to each employee, reviewed and updated on an annual basis, and considered a written protocol for the office.**

24. When an employee has a needlestick injury the employee should

   d. **all of the above – OSHA requires the employer to offer all of the above options, such as accepting blood testing for HIV and HBV at recommended intervals, having the HBV gamma globulin administered as soon as possible at no cost to the employee, and documenting the incident with the office manager.**

25. Part of the hazard communication protocol includes

   d. **all of the above.**

26. According to the American Heart Association, cardiopulmonary resuscitation certification should be updated

   b. **every 2 years.**

27. OSHA considers Category 1 workers as those who

   d. **come into contact with blood and body fluids or tissues.**

28. OSHA states that Category 3 workers

   a. **are not exposed to blood or bodily fluids.**

29. After an exposure incident, according to the blood-borne pathogens standard, an employer must keep a log that includes

   d. **all of the above – Location of the incident, description of how it happened, and what type of follow-up care was taken are all steps taken after an exposure incident.**

30. According to OSHA, employee training records relating to the Bloodborne and Hazard Communication Standard must be maintained for a minimum of

   c. **3 years.**

31. Who provides the SDS sheets that are required to be kept in the dental office?

   c. **chemical manufacturer – They either come with the product or should be requested.**

32. The letters CDC stand for

   d. **Centers for Disease Control.**

33. The standard that is created to protect employees against occupational exposure to blood-borne, disease-causing organisms is referred to as which standard?

   a. **OSHA Bloodborne Pathogens Standard – This standard emphasizes that all people are potentially infectious.**

34. Which of the following is a work practice control?

   a. **hand washing following glove removal. – All the other examples are engineering controls.**

35. Which of the following is an engineering control?

   b. **self-sheathing needles – All the others are work practice controls.**

Chapter 1: General Chairside Assisting

Section I: Collection and Recording of Clinical Data

DIRECTIONS: Darken the space under the selected answer.

	A	B	C	D			A	B	C	D
1.	❑	❑	❑	❑		23.	❑	❑	❑	❑
2.	❑	❑	❑	❑		24.	❑	❑	❑	❑
3.	❑	❑	❑	❑		25.	❑	❑	❑	❑
4.	❑	❑	❑	❑		26.	❑	❑	❑	❑
5.	❑	❑	❑	❑		27.	❑	❑	❑	❑
6.	❑	❑	❑	❑		28.	❑	❑	❑	❑
7.	❑	❑	❑	❑		29.	❑	❑	❑	❑
8.	❑	❑	❑	❑		30.	❑	❑	❑	❑
9.	❑	❑	❑	❑		31.	❑	❑	❑	❑
10.	❑	❑	❑	❑		32.	❑	❑	❑	❑
11.	❑	❑	❑	❑		33.	❑	❑	❑	❑
12.	❑	❑	❑	❑		34.	❑	❑	❑	❑
13.	❑	❑	❑	❑		35.	❑	❑	❑	❑
14.	❑	❑	❑	❑		36.	❑	❑	❑	❑
15.	❑	❑	❑	❑		37.	❑	❑	❑	❑
16.	❑	❑	❑	❑		38.	❑	❑	❑	❑
17.	❑	❑	❑	❑		39.	❑	❑	❑	❑
18.	❑	❑	❑	❑		40.	❑	❑	❑	❑
19.	❑	❑	❑	❑		41.	❑	❑	❑	❑
20.	❑	❑	❑	❑		42.	❑	❑	❑	❑
21.	❑	❑	❑	❑		43.	❑	❑	❑	❑
22.	❑	❑	❑	❑		44.	❑	❑	❑	❑

	A	B	C	D			A	B	C	D
45.	❑	❑	❑	❑		60.	❑	❑	❑	❑
46.	❑	❑	❑	❑		61.	❑	❑	❑	❑
47.	❑	❑	❑	❑		62.	❑	❑	❑	❑
48.	❑	❑	❑	❑		63.	❑	❑	❑	❑
49.	❑	❑	❑	❑		64.	❑	❑	❑	❑
50.	❑	❑	❑	❑		65.	❑	❑	❑	❑
51.	❑	❑	❑	❑		66.	❑	❑	❑	❑
52.	❑	❑	❑	❑		67.	❑	❑	❑	❑
53.	❑	❑	❑	❑		68.	❑	❑	❑	❑
54.	❑	❑	❑	❑		69.	❑	❑	❑	❑
55.	❑	❑	❑	❑		70.	❑	❑	❑	❑
56.	❑	❑	❑	❑		71.	❑	❑	❑	❑
57.	❑	❑	❑	❑		72.	❑	❑	❑	❑
58.	❑	❑	❑	❑		73.	❑	❑	❑	❑
59.	❑	❑	❑	❑						

Section II: Chairside Dental Procedures

DIRECTIONS: Darken the space under the selected answer.

	A	B	C	D			A	B	C	D
1.	❑	❑	❑	❑		13.	❑	❑	❑	❑
2.	❑	❑	❑	❑		14.	❑	❑	❑	❑
3.	❑	❑	❑	❑		15.	❑	❑	❑	❑
4.	❑	❑	❑	❑		16.	❑	❑	❑	❑
5.	❑	❑	❑	❑		17.	❑	❑	❑	❑
6.	❑	❑	❑	❑		18.	❑	❑	❑	❑
7.	❑	❑	❑	❑		19.	❑	❑	❑	❑
8.	❑	❑	❑	❑		20.	❑	❑	❑	❑
9.	❑	❑	❑	❑		21.	❑	❑	❑	❑
10.	❑	❑	❑	❑		22.	❑	❑	❑	❑
11.	❑	❑	❑	❑		23.	❑	❑	❑	❑
12.	❑	❑	❑	❑		24.	❑	❑	❑	❑

	A	B	C	D			A	B	C	D
25.	❏	❏	❏	❏		43.	❏	❏	❏	❏
26.	❏	❏	❏	❏		44.	❏	❏	❏	❏
27.	❏	❏	❏	❏		45.	❏	❏	❏	❏
28.	❏	❏	❏	❏		46.	❏	❏	❏	❏
29.	❏	❏	❏	❏		47.	❏	❏	❏	❏
30.	❏	❏	❏	❏		48.	❏	❏	❏	❏
31.	❏	❏	❏	❏		49.	❏	❏	❏	❏
32.	❏	❏	❏	❏		50.	❏	❏	❏	❏
33.	❏	❏	❏	❏		51.	❏	❏	❏	❏
34.	❏	❏	❏	❏		52.	❏	❏	❏	❏
35.	❏	❏	❏	❏		53.	❏	❏	❏	❏
36.	❏	❏	❏	❏		54.	❏	❏	❏	❏
37.	❏	❏	❏	❏		55.	❏	❏	❏	❏
38.	❏	❏	❏	❏		56.	❏	❏	❏	❏
39.	❏	❏	❏	❏		57.	❏	❏	❏	❏
40.	❏	❏	❏	❏		58.	❏	❏	❏	❏
41.	❏	❏	❏	❏		59.	❏	❏	❏	❏
42.	❏	❏	❏	❏						

Section III: Chairside Dental Materials
(Preparation, Manipulation, Application)

DIRECTIONS: Darken the space under the selected answer.

	A	B	C	D			A	B	C	D
1.	❏	❏	❏	❏		9.	❏	❏	❏	❏
2.	❏	❏	❏	❏		10.	❏	❏	❏	❏
3.	❏	❏	❏	❏		11.	❏	❏	❏	❏
4.	❏	❏	❏	❏		12.	❏	❏	❏	❏
5.	❏	❏	❏	❏		13.	❏	❏	❏	❏
6.	❏	❏	❏	❏		14.	❏	❏	❏	❏
7.	❏	❏	❏	❏		15.	❏	❏	❏	❏
8.	❏	❏	❏	❏		16.	❏	❏	❏	❏

	A	B	C	D			A	B	C	D
17.	❏	❏	❏	❏		20.	❏	❏	❏	❏
18.	❏	❏	❏	❏		21.	❏	❏	❏	❏
19.	❏	❏	❏	❏		22.	❏	❏	❏	❏

Section IV: Lab Materials and Procedures

DIRECTIONS: Darken the space under the selected answer.

	A	B	C	D			A	B	C	D
1.	❏	❏	❏	❏		9.	❏	❏	❏	❏
2.	❏	❏	❏	❏		10.	❏	❏	❏	❏
3.	❏	❏	❏	❏		11.	❏	❏	❏	❏
4.	❏	❏	❏	❏		12.	❏	❏	❏	❏
5.	❏	❏	❏	❏		13.	❏	❏	❏	❏
6.	❏	❏	❏	❏		14.	❏	❏	❏	❏
7.	❏	❏	❏	❏		15.	❏	❏	❏	❏
8.	❏	❏	❏	❏		16.	❏	❏	❏	❏

Section V: Patient Education and Oral Health Management

DIRECTIONS: Darken the space under the selected answer.

	A	B	C	D			A	B	C	D
1.	❏	❏	❏	❏		12.	❏	❏	❏	❏
2.	❏	❏	❏	❏		13.	❏	❏	❏	❏
3.	❏	❏	❏	❏		14.	❏	❏	❏	❏
4.	❏	❏	❏	❏		15.	❏	❏	❏	❏
5.	❏	❏	❏	❏		16.	❏	❏	❏	❏
6.	❏	❏	❏	❏		17.	❏	❏	❏	❏
7.	❏	❏	❏	❏		18.	❏	❏	❏	❏
8.	❏	❏	❏	❏		19.	❏	❏	❏	❏
9.	❏	❏	❏	❏		20.	❏	❏	❏	❏
10.	❏	❏	❏	❏		21.	❏	❏	❏	❏
11.	❏	❏	❏	❏		22.	❏	❏	❏	❏

	A	B	C	D			A	B	C	D
23.	❑	❑	❑	❑		27.	❑	❑	❑	❑
24.	❑	❑	❑	❑		28.	❑	❑	❑	❑
25.	❑	❑	❑	❑		29.	❑	❑	❑	❑
26.	❑	❑	❑	❑						

Section VI: Prevention and Management of Emergencies

DIRECTIONS: Darken the space under the selected answer.

	A	B	C	D			A	B	C	D
1.	❑	❑	❑	❑		14.	❑	❑	❑	❑
2.	❑	❑	❑	❑		15.	❑	❑	❑	❑
3.	❑	❑	❑	❑		16.	❑	❑	❑	❑
4.	❑	❑	❑	❑		17.	❑	❑	❑	❑
5.	❑	❑	❑	❑		18.	❑	❑	❑	❑
6.	❑	❑	❑	❑		19.	❑	❑	❑	❑
7.	❑	❑	❑	❑		20.	❑	❑	❑	❑
8.	❑	❑	❑	❑		21.	❑	❑	❑	❑
9.	❑	❑	❑	❑		22.	❑	❑	❑	❑
10.	❑	❑	❑	❑		23.	❑	❑	❑	❑
11.	❑	❑	❑	❑		24.	❑	❑	❑	❑
12.	❑	❑	❑	❑		25.	❑	❑	❑	❑
13.	❑	❑	❑	❑						

Section VII: Office Operations

DIRECTIONS: Darken the space under the selected answer.

	A	B	C	D			A	B	C	D
1.	❑	❑	❑	❑		7.	❑	❑	❑	❑
2.	❑	❑	❑	❑		8.	❑	❑	❑	❑
3.	❑	❑	❑	❑		9.	❑	❑	❑	❑
4.	❑	❑	❑	❑		10.	❑	❑	❑	❑
5.	❑	❑	❑	❑		11.	❑	❑	❑	❑
6.	❑	❑	❑	❑		12.	❑	❑	❑	❑

	A	B	C	D		A	B	C	D
13.	❑	❑	❑	❑	19.	❑	❑	❑	❑
14.	❑	❑	❑	❑	20.	❑	❑	❑	❑
15.	❑	❑	❑	❑	21.	❑	❑	❑	❑
16.	❑	❑	❑	❑	22.	❑	❑	❑	❑
17.	❑	❑	❑	❑	23.	❑	❑	❑	❑
18.	❑	❑	❑	❑					

Chapter 2: Radiation Health and Safety

Section I: Expose and Evaluate

DIRECTIONS: Darken the space under the selected answer.

	A	B	C	D			A	B	C	D
1.	❏	❏	❏	❏		28.	❏	❏	❏	❏
2.	❏	❏	❏	❏		29.	❏	❏	❏	❏
3.	❏	❏	❏	❏		30.	❏	❏	❏	❏
4.	❏	❏	❏	❏		31.	❏	❏	❏	❏
5.	❏	❏	❏	❏		32.	❏	❏	❏	❏
6.	❏	❏	❏	❏		33.	❏	❏	❏	❏
7.	❏	❏	❏	❏		34.	❏	❏	❏	❏
8.	❏	❏	❏	❏		35.	❏	❏	❏	❏
9.	❏	❏	❏	❏		36.	❏	❏	❏	❏
10.	❏	❏	❏	❏		37.	❏	❏	❏	❏
11.	❏	❏	❏	❏		38.	❏	❏	❏	❏
12.	❏	❏	❏	❏		39.	❏	❏	❏	❏
13.	❏	❏	❏	❏		40.	❏	❏	❏	❏
14.	❏	❏	❏	❏		41.	❏	❏	❏	❏
15.	❏	❏	❏	❏		42.	❏	❏	❏	❏
16.	❏	❏	❏	❏		43.	❏	❏	❏	❏
17.	❏	❏	❏	❏		44.	❏	❏	❏	❏
18.	❏	❏	❏	❏		45.	❏	❏	❏	❏
19.	❏	❏	❏	❏		46.	❏	❏	❏	❏
20.	❏	❏	❏	❏		47.	❏	❏	❏	❏
21.	❏	❏	❏	❏		48.	❏	❏	❏	❏
22.	❏	❏	❏	❏		49.	❏	❏	❏	❏
23.	❏	❏	❏	❏		50.	❏	❏	❏	❏
24.	❏	❏	❏	❏		51.	❏	❏	❏	❏
25.	❏	❏	❏	❏		52.	❏	❏	❏	❏
26.	❏	❏	❏	❏		53.	❏	❏	❏	❏
27.	❏	❏	❏	❏		54.	❏	❏	❏	❏

	A	B	C	D			A	B	C	D
55.	❏	❏	❏	❏		82.	❏	❏	❏	❏
56.	❏	❏	❏	❏		83.	❏	❏	❏	❏
57.	❏	❏	❏	❏		84.	❏	❏	❏	❏
58.	❏	❏	❏	❏		85.	❏	❏	❏	❏
59.	❏	❏	❏	❏		86.	❏	❏	❏	❏
60.	❏	❏	❏	❏		87.	❏	❏	❏	❏
61.	❏	❏	❏	❏		88.	❏	❏	❏	❏
62.	❏	❏	❏	❏		89.	❏	❏	❏	❏
63.	❏	❏	❏	❏		90.	❏	❏	❏	❏
64.	❏	❏	❏	❏		91.	❏	❏	❏	❏
65.	❏	❏	❏	❏		92.	❏	❏	❏	❏
66.	❏	❏	❏	❏		93.	❏	❏	❏	❏
67.	❏	❏	❏	❏		94.	❏	❏	❏	❏
68.	❏	❏	❏	❏		95.	❏	❏	❏	❏
69.	❏	❏	❏	❏		96.	❏	❏	❏	❏
70.	❏	❏	❏	❏		97.	❏	❏	❏	❏
71.	❏	❏	❏	❏		99.	❏	❏	❏	❏
72.	❏	❏	❏	❏		100.	❏	❏	❏	❏
73.	❏	❏	❏	❏		101.	❏	❏	❏	❏
74.	❏	❏	❏	❏		102.	❏	❏	❏	❏
75.	❏	❏	❏	❏		103.	❏	❏	❏	❏
76.	❏	❏	❏	❏		104.	❏	❏	❏	❏
77.	❏	❏	❏	❏		105.	❏	❏	❏	❏
78.	❏	❏	❏	❏		106.	❏	❏	❏	❏
79.	❏	❏	❏	❏		107.	❏	❏	❏	❏
80.	❏	❏	❏	❏		108.	❏	❏	❏	❏
81.	❏	❏	❏	❏		109.	❏	❏	❏	❏

Section II: Quality Assurance and Radiology Regulations

DIRECTIONS: Darken the space under the selected answer.

	A	B	C	D			A	B	C	D
1.	❏	❏	❏	❏		18.	❏	❏	❏	❏
2.	❏	❏	❏	❏		19.	❏	❏	❏	❏
3.	❏	❏	❏	❏		20.	❏	❏	❏	❏
4.	❏	❏	❏	❏		21.	❏	❏	❏	❏
5.	❏	❏	❏	❏		22.	❏	❏	❏	❏
6.	❏	❏	❏	❏		23.	❏	❏	❏	❏
7.	❏	❏	❏	❏		24.	❏	❏	❏	❏
8.	❏	❏	❏	❏		25.	❏	❏	❏	❏
9.	❏	❏	❏	❏		26.	❏	❏	❏	❏
10.	❏	❏	❏	❏		27.	❏	❏	❏	❏
11.	❏	❏	❏	❏		28.	❏	❏	❏	❏
12.	❏	❏	❏	❏		29.	❏	❏	❏	❏
13.	❏	❏	❏	❏		30.	❏	❏	❏	❏
14.	❏	❏	❏	❏		31.	❏	❏	❏	❏
15.	❏	❏	❏	❏		32.	❏	❏	❏	❏
16.	❏	❏	❏	❏		33.	❏	❏	❏	❏
17.	❏	❏	❏	❏						

Section III: Radiation Safety for Patients and Operators

DIRECTIONS: Darken the space under the selected answer.

	A	B	C	D			A	B	C	D
1.	❏	❏	❏	❏		9.	❏	❏	❏	❏
2.	❏	❏	❏	❏		10.	❏	❏	❏	❏
3.	❏	❏	❏	❏		11.	❏	❏	❏	❏
4.	❏	❏	❏	❏		12.	❏	❏	❏	❏
5.	❏	❏	❏	❏		13.	❏	❏	❏	❏
6.	❏	❏	❏	❏		14.	❏	❏	❏	❏
7.	❏	❏	❏	❏		15.	❏	❏	❏	❏
8.	❏	❏	❏	❏		16.	❏	❏	❏	❏

	A	B	C	D			A	B	C	D
17.	❏	❏	❏	❏		43.	❏	❏	❏	❏
18.	❏	❏	❏	❏		44.	❏	❏	❏	❏
19.	❏	❏	❏	❏		45.	❏	❏	❏	❏
20.	❏	❏	❏	❏		46.	❏	❏	❏	❏
21.	❏	❏	❏	❏		47.	❏	❏	❏	❏
22.	❏	❏	❏	❏		48.	❏	❏	❏	❏
23.	❏	❏	❏	❏		49.	❏	❏	❏	❏
24.	❏	❏	❏	❏		50.	❏	❏	❏	❏
25.	❏	❏	❏	❏		51.	❏	❏	❏	❏
26.	❏	❏	❏	❏		52.	❏	❏	❏	❏
27.	❏	❏	❏	❏		53.	❏	❏	❏	❏
28.	❏	❏	❏	❏		54.	❏	❏	❏	❏
29.	❏	❏	❏	❏		55.	❏	❏	❏	❏
30.	❏	❏	❏	❏		56.	❏	❏	❏	❏
31.	❏	❏	❏	❏		57.	❏	❏	❏	❏
32.	❏	❏	❏	❏		58.	❏	❏	❏	❏
33.	❏	❏	❏	❏		59.	❏	❏	❏	❏
34.	❏	❏	❏	❏		60.	❏	❏	❏	❏
35.	❏	❏	❏	❏		61.	❏	❏	❏	❏
36.	❏	❏	❏	❏		62.	❏	❏	❏	❏
37.	❏	❏	❏	❏		63.	❏	❏	❏	❏
38.	❏	❏	❏	❏		64.	❏	❏	❏	❏
39.	❏	❏	❏	❏		65.	❏	❏	❏	❏
40.	❏	❏	❏	❏		66.	❏	❏	❏	❏
41.	❏	❏	❏	❏		67.	❏	❏	❏	❏
42.	❏	❏	❏	❏		68.	❏	❏	❏	❏

Section IV: Infection Control

DIRECTIONS: Darken the space under the selected answer.

	A	B	C	D			A	B	C	D
1.	❏	❏	❏	❏		12.	❏	❏	❏	❏
2.	❏	❏	❏	❏		13.	❏	❏	❏	❏
3.	❏	❏	❏	❏		14.	❏	❏	❏	❏
4.	❏	❏	❏	❏		15.	❏	❏	❏	❏
5.	❏	❏	❏	❏		16.	❏	❏	❏	❏
6.	❏	❏	❏	❏		17.	❏	❏	❏	❏
7.	❏	❏	❏	❏		18.	❏	❏	❏	❏
8.	❏	❏	❏	❏		19.	❏	❏	❏	❏
9.	❏	❏	❏	❏		20.	❏	❏	❏	❏
10.	❏	❏	❏	❏		21.	❏	❏	❏	❏
11.	❏	❏	❏	❏						

Chapter 3: Infection Control

Section 1: Patient and Dental Health Care Worker Education

DIRECTIONS: Darken the space under the selected answer.

	A	B	C	D			A	B	C	D
1.	❑	❑	❑	❑		14.	❑	❑	❑	❑
2.	❑	❑	❑	❑		15.	❑	❑	❑	❑
3.	❑	❑	❑	❑		16.	❑	❑	❑	❑
4.	❑	❑	❑	❑		17.	❑	❑	❑	❑
5.	❑	❑	❑	❑		18.	❑	❑	❑	❑
6.	❑	❑	❑	❑		19.	❑	❑	❑	❑
7.	❑	❑	❑	❑		20.	❑	❑	❑	❑
8.	❑	❑	❑	❑		21.	❑	❑	❑	❑
9.	❑	❑	❑	❑		22.	❑	❑	❑	❑
10.	❑	❑	❑	❑		23.	❑	❑	❑	❑
11.	❑	❑	❑	❑		24.	❑	❑	❑	❑
12.	❑	❑	❑	❑		25.	❑	❑	❑	❑
13.	❑	❑	❑	❑						

Section II: Standard/Universal Precautions and the Prevention of Disease Transmission

DIRECTIONS: Darken the space under the selected answer.

	A	B	C	D			A	B	C	D
1.	❑	❑	❑	❑		9.	❑	❑	❑	❑
2.	❑	❑	❑	❑		10.	❑	❑	❑	❑
3.	❑	❑	❑	❑		11.	❑	❑	❑	❑
4.	❑	❑	❑	❑		12.	❑	❑	❑	❑
5.	❑	❑	❑	❑		13.	❑	❑	❑	❑
6.	❑	❑	❑	❑		14.	❑	❑	❑	❑
7.	❑	❑	❑	❑		15.	❑	❑	❑	❑
8.	❑	❑	❑	❑		16.	❑	❑	❑	❑

	A	B	C	D			A	B	C	D
17.	❑	❑	❑	❑		47.	❑	❑	❑	❑
18.	❑	❑	❑	❑		48.	❑	❑	❑	❑
19.	❑	❑	❑	❑		49.	❑	❑	❑	❑
20.	❑	❑	❑	❑		50.	❑	❑	❑	❑
21.	❑	❑	❑	❑		51.	❑	❑	❑	❑
22.	❑	❑	❑	❑		52.	❑	❑	❑	❑
23.	❑	❑	❑	❑		53.	❑	❑	❑	❑
24.	❑	❑	❑	❑		54.	❑	❑	❑	❑
25.	❑	❑	❑	❑		55.	❑	❑	❑	❑
26.	❑	❑	❑	❑		56.	❑	❑	❑	❑
27.	❑	❑	❑	❑		57.	❑	❑	❑	❑
28.	❑	❑	❑	❑		58.	❑	❑	❑	❑
29.	❑	❑	❑	❑		59.	❑	❑	❑	❑
30.	❑	❑	❑	❑		60.	❑	❑	❑	❑
31.	❑	❑	❑	❑		61.	❑	❑	❑	❑
32.	❑	❑	❑	❑		62.	❑	❑	❑	❑
33.	❑	❑	❑	❑		63.	❑	❑	❑	❑
34.	❑	❑	❑	❑		64.	❑	❑	❑	❑
35.	❑	❑	❑	❑		65.	❑	❑	❑	❑
36.	❑	❑	❑	❑		66.	❑	❑	❑	❑
37.	❑	❑	❑	❑		67.	❑	❑	❑	❑
38.	❑	❑	❑	❑		68.	❑	❑	❑	❑
39.	❑	❑	❑	❑		69.	❑	❑	❑	❑
40.	❑	❑	❑	❑		70.	❑	❑	❑	❑
41.	❑	❑	❑	❑		71.	❑	❑	❑	❑
42.	❑	❑	❑	❑		72.	❑	❑	❑	❑
43.	❑	❑	❑	❑		73.	❑	❑	❑	❑
44.	❑	❑	❑	❑		74.	❑	❑	❑	❑
45.	❑	❑	❑	❑		75.	❑	❑	❑	❑
46.	❑	❑	❑	❑						

Section III: Occupational Safety

DIRECTIONS: Darken the space under the selected answer.

	A	B	C	D		A	B	C	D
1.	❏	❏	❏	❏	19.	❏	❏	❏	❏
2.	❏	❏	❏	❏	20.	❏	❏	❏	❏
3.	❏	❏	❏	❏	21.	❏	❏	❏	❏
4.	❏	❏	❏	❏	22.	❏	❏	❏	❏
5.	❏	❏	❏	❏	23.	❏	❏	❏	❏
6.	❏	❏	❏	❏	24.	❏	❏	❏	❏
7.	❏	❏	❏	❏	25.	❏	❏	❏	❏
8.	❏	❏	❏	❏	26.	❏	❏	❏	❏
9.	❏	❏	❏	❏	27.	❏	❏	❏	❏
10.	❏	❏	❏	❏	28.	❏	❏	❏	❏
11.	❏	❏	❏	❏	29.	❏	❏	❏	❏
12.	❏	❏	❏	❏	30.	❏	❏	❏	❏
13.	❏	❏	❏	❏	31.	❏	❏	❏	❏
14.	❏	❏	❏	❏	32.	❏	❏	❏	❏
15.	❏	❏	❏	❏	33.	❏	❏	❏	❏
16.	❏	❏	❏	❏	34.	❏	❏	❏	❏
17.	❏	❏	❏	❏	35.	❏	❏	❏	❏
18.	❏	❏	❏	❏					

INDEX

Page numbers followed by "f" indicate figures.

equipment
    considerations for managing, 94–95
    laboratory, 61
    maintenance, 79–80
    for radiographic technique, 89–91
    single-use disposable, 152–153
    standard precautions for, 137
    for sterilization, 157
eruption of teeth, 65
etchants, 53, 55
exfoliation of teeth, 64–65
existing conditions, dental charting, 16
exposure control plan, 174, 178f
exposure incident, 170, 174
exposure time, radiography, 126
external pterygoid (lateral) muscle, 3–4
extraction tray, 37, 37f
extraoral radiographs, 88
eye protection, 176f

F

facial bones, 2–3, 2f
facial expression, muscles of, 4–5, 4f
facial nerve, 6
facial surface of teeth, 15
fast film, 125–126
fecal-oral route transmission, 143
filiform papillae, tongue, 12
film artifact on radiograph, 98, 98f
film badge, 125, 128
film bending on radiograph, 102, 102f
film cassettes, radiograph, 93
film density, radiographic exposure, 91
film distortion, 95, 96f
film packets, radiograph
    parts and functions of, 93, 93f
    purpose of, 91
film placement errors on radiograph, 102
film speed, radiographic exposure, 91, 128
film-holding devices, 89, 90f
filter, 125–126
filtration, radiographic exposure, 91, 125–126
fingerprints on radiograph, 101, 101f
fixer, 88, 95, 156
fluoride, 64, 67
fluoride application tray, 38
fogged film on radiograph, 99, 100f
foliate papillae, tongue, 12
foreshortening on radiograph, 96, 96f
four-handed dentistry techniques, 31–34, 32f
    with restorative procedures, 44

free gingiva, 11
frenum, 1, 11
frontalis muscle, 4
fungiform papillae, tongue, 12

G

glands and lymphatics, 5–6
glass ionomer cements, 53–55
glossopharyngeal nerve, 6
gloves, occupational safety, 176f
gypsum products, 60

H

hand hygiene techniques, 152
hard palate, 1, 11
hazard communication program, 174
Hazard Communication Standard, OSHA, 118–119, 170
    first aid procedures, 171
    orientation, 171
    requirements, 174
healing process, systemic disease on, 66
Health Insurance Portability and Accountability Act (HIPAA), 81
hepatitis, 143–145
hepatitis A virus (HAV), 143, 144
hepatitis B vaccination, 177f
hepatitis B virus (HBV), 143, 144
hepatitis C virus (HCV), 143, 144
hepatitis D virus (HDV), 144
hepatitis E virus (HEV), 144, 145
herpes, 143, 145
herringbone effect, 99, 99f
high-level chemical germicides, sterilization, 157
horizontal overlapping on radiograph, 96, 97f
hospital disinfectant, 160
housekeeping, quality-assurance program, 173–174, 176f
HSV, 145
HSV 1, 145
HSV 2, 145
human immunodeficiency virus (HIV), 143, 145
hyperventilation, 14, 73
hypoglossal nerve, 6
hypotension, 73

I

identification dot, 88, 103
immunization, 143
    against infectious disease, 147
impactions, tray setup, 39

factors influencing quality, 91–92

infection control techniques, 137

patient positioning during, 93–94

reasons for retaining and, 119

radiographic film. *See also* radiograph film packets

conditions for film processing, 118–119

selecting, 89

storage area, 118

radiographic images, errors

acquiring, 95–99

exposing panoramic radiographs, 102–103

improper handling of, 101–102

processing, 99–101

radiographic technique

equipment for, 89–91

selecting, 88–89

radiographs

for diagnostic value, 95–103

methods for duplicating, 119

mounting and labeling, 103–104

radiology regulations, 119–120

radiolucent, 88, 104

radiopaque, 88, 100, 104

regulated waste, 170, 173

replenisher, 88, 95

respiration, 14

restorative materials, dental, 54

reticulation on radiograph, 101

reversible hydrocolloid (agar-gar) material, 53

RHS (Radiation Health and Safety), 87–141

RHS, expose and evaluate, 87–117

acquiring radiographic images, 91–94

answers and rationales, 113–117

conventional film processing, 95

digital radiography, 94–95

equipment for radiographic technique, 89–91

mounting and labeling radiographs, 103–104

patient management, 104

patient preparation for radiographic
exposures, 88

radiographs for diagnostic value, 92–103

review questions, 106–112

selecting radiographic technique, 88–89

RHS, infection control for

answers and rationales, 141

review questions, 139–140

standard precautions for equipment, 137

standard precautions for patients/operators, 137

RHS, quality assurance, 118–119

answers and rationales, 123–124

and radiology regulations, 119–120

review questions, 121–122

Rinn device, 89, 90f, 94

root planning and curettage, tray setup, 41

rotary instruments, tray setup, 41

routine radiographs, 127

rubber dams, 154

rugae, 12

S

safelights, 118–119

Safety Data Sheet (SDS), 160

saliva, functions of, 66

salivary glands and ducts, 5–6, 5f

scatter radiation, 125–126, 127f

scope and application, occupational safety, 175f

scratched film on radiograph, 101

sealant application, tray setup, 41, 42f

secondary radiation, 125–126, 127f

sedative dressing, 53, 55

sedative/palliative materials, dental, 54–55

semicritical items, 161

severe acute respiratory syndrome (SARS), 145

sharps, 152, 155, 155f, 170, 173, 175f

shelf life, 118

shielding, 126

shock, 73–74

short-term effects of x-radiation, 127

single-handed transfer technique, 33, 33f

single-use disposable materials/equipment, 152–153

sinus, 88–89, 104

six-handed transfer technique, 34

Snap-A-Rays, 89, 90f, 94, 158

soft palate, 1, 11

spleen, 6

spore testing, 159

spotted film on radiograph, 100, 100f

spray-wipe-spray method, 159

stainless steel crown placement/removal, tray setup, 42, 42f

standard precautions

for equipment, 137

for patients/operators, 137

standard/universal precautions and prevention of disease transmission answers and rationales, 167–169

asepsis procedures, 159–161

cross-contamination and, 152–154

instrument processing, 157–159

maintaining aseptic conditions, 154–156

review questions, 162–166

State Dental Practice Act, 79, 81

static electricity artifacts on radiograph, 101

static zone, 31–32
sterilization, 152, 156–161
    autoclave, 158
    chemclave, 158
    cold, 158
    disinfectant comparisons, 157
    dry heat, 158
    high-level chemical germicides, 157
    instruments and equipment for, 157
    intermediate-level chemical germicides, 157
    low-level chemical germicides, 157
    methods for, 157–158
sublingual gland, 6
submandibular gland, 6
succedaneous teeth, 64–65
supernumerary teeth, 88–89
supply and inventory control, 79
suture placement and removal, tray setup, 42–43
syncope, 73–74
systemic diseases
    effects on healing process, 66
    oral manifestations of, 14
systolic blood pressure, 14, 73

T

teeth/tooth, 10, 11f
    desensitization tray setup, 36
    divisions of, 10
    eruption and exfoliation of, 65
    structure, 10
    succedaneous, 64–65
    surfaces of, 15, 15f
    views, 103
temporalis muscle, 3
temporary cementation tray setup, 42
temporary restoration tray setup, 43
temporary restorative materials, 54
tetanus infection, 146
thymus gland, 6
tongue, 11–12, 12f
tonsils, 6, 12
    location of, 13f
torn film on radiograph, 101
training components, occupational safety, 177f
training records, 174, 178f
transfer zone, 31–32
tray setups, armamentaria, 34–43
    amalgam restoration, 35, 35f
    anesthetic, 34, 34f
    composite restorations, 35, 35f
    crown and bridge preparation/cementation, 36, 36f

dental dam, 38, 38f
endodontic therapy, 37, 37f
extraction, 37, 37f
fluoride application, 38
immediate dentures, 39
impactions, 39
implants, 39, 39f
incision and drainage, 38
initial/secondary impressions, 40
interceptive orthodontics, 40
occlusal equilibration/adjustment, 40, 40f
oral examination, 40
oral prophylaxis, 40, 41f
periodontal procedures, 41
periodontal surgical dressing placement/
    removal, 41
removable partial/full denture fabrication,
    38, 38f
root planning and curettage, 41
rotary instruments, 41
sealant application, 41, 42f
stainless steel crown placement/removal,
    42, 42f
suture placement and removal, 42–43
tooth desensitization, 36
treatment documentation, 21, 22f
trigeminal nerve, 6
    mandibular branch of, 6, 8f
    maxillary branch of, 6, 7f
tuberculosis (TB), 145
two-handed transfer technique, 34, 34f

U

underexposed film on radiograph, 98, 98f
Universal Numbering System, 15, 15f
universal precautions, 170, 173
uvula, 11

V

varnishes, 54
vector-borne transmission, 154, 155
vehicle transmission, 154, 155
veins, 9, 10f

W

waste handling, 173, 176f
waste materials, disposal of, 155–156
waxes, dental, 53, 60
white lines on radiograph, 101

whitening agents, 55
work practice control, 170, 173, 175f

X

xerostomia (dry mouth), 64, 66
x-rays, 95, 125, 129
    factors affecting production, 126

machine factors influencing radiation safety, 126
machine malfunctions, 126–127
x-radiation biology, 127–129
x-radiation physics, 126, 127f, 128–129

Z

zygomatic major muscle, 5